DASH Diet Cookbook

Decrease Blood Pressure Naturally with Delicious Everyday Recipes

Jennifer Stone

medical or professional advice. The content within this book has been derived from various sources. Please consult a licensed professional before attempting any techniques outlined in this book.

By reading this document, the reader agrees that under no circumstances are is the author responsible for any losses, direct or indirect, which are incurred as a result of the use of information contained within this document, including, but not limited to errors, omissions, or inaccuracies.

Table Of Contents

Introduction – What Is a DASH Diet, and Why Is It Healthy?

DASH is short for Dietary Approaches to Stop Hypertension.

People who desire a control over their hypertension are recommended the DASH diet. Hypertension is a condition of HBP (high blood pressure) in a person. A consistent struggle with high blood pressure can usually lead to heart diseases, which is why the DASH diet becomes an extremely important solution for people.

In the DASH diet plan, a person focuses on a combination of nutritious ingredients, such as whole grains, lean meats, vegetables, and fruits. Lean meat protein includes fish and chicken; however, vegans or vegetarians can choose beans in order to get lean protein. This diet plan reduces the amount of red meat, added sugars, fat and salt in meals. These are the ingredients that provide threats of hypertension in the human body.

There are a variety of reasons why the DASH diet is considered a healthy dietary plan for people:

1. The DASH Diet Decreases the Risk of Cancer

By reducing HBP in a person's body, this dietary plan helps in the reduction of cancer threats. People, who avoid red meat, salt, and added sugars, and stick to a DASH diet, are more protected from colorectal cancer and breast cancer as well.

2. The DASH Diet Helps in Losing Weight

This dietary plan cuts out a lot of sugary food options, high-fat and other harmful ingredients that make people lose control of their own body weight. Cutting harmful food choices allows people to stick to vegetables, whole grains, fruits and lean protein. Consistently following such food habits results in losing weight for sure, but you have to control the calorie intake on a daily basis. Your body should get lesser calories than it is burning every day.

3. The DASH Diet Reduces the Risk of Metabolic Syndrome

Metabolic syndrome includes a variety of conditions that result in cardiovascular and diabetes diseases. These syndrome conditions are induced due to high-fat diets and the presence of too much red meat in your food; hence, changing your diet to DASH creates better metabolic health in your body, providing safety from the metabolic syndrome.

4. The DASH Diet Reduces Your Risk of Diabetes

If your family has a history of diabetes, you have to take care of your diet even before the signs appear in your physical health. This dietary plan is suitable for every person who wants protection from diabetes. Insulin resistance is improved with this dietary habit, which protects from the development of type 2 diabetes in your body.

5. The DASH Diet Saves You from Heart Problems

Heart disease is the ultimate outcome of high blood pressure. If you don't control your high BP levels with your diet, it turns into severe heart issues. In fact, the risk of heart stroke increases due to high blood pressure.

Shifting to a blood pressure-friendly diet, your heart gets protection from the hypertension issues. More vegetables and fruit content in your diet create a safer nutritional intake for your body that doesn't trigger heart problems.

CHAPTER 1 – The Science Behind a DASH Diet

In our body, the stream of blood in our blood vessels results in a pressure force on the vessels as well as the organs. There are two types of pressures that the blood flow creates in our body:

1. Diastolic Pressure

Between two heartbeats, our heart stays at rest. During this time, the blood flow puts all the pressure on the blood vessels. This pressure is called Diastolic Pressure in the human body.

2. Systolic Pressure

When our heart beats, the blood flow transfers a pressure to the vessels. This pressure is called the Systolic Pressure.

For a healthy adult, the diastolic pressure should be lower than 80 mmHg; plus, the systolic pressure should be lower than 120 mmHg. In a blood pressure reading, this calculation is introduced as: 120/80. If this reading crosses the limit and becomes 140/90, the person could be diagnosed as having hypertension.

The science behind the DASH diet is simple. It contains ingredients that reduce blood pressure in a person's body, or, it can be said that the DASH diet removes all the HBP-inducing ingredients from a person's diet.

When aligned with a controlled calorie intake, the DASH diet also helps in reducing body weight. The diet follower stops consuming too much salt or red meat in the diet, so the body starts burning calories easily without putting pressure on the metabolic system.

The Magic of Sodium Reduction in Your Diet

As the DASH diet is all about fruits, vegetables, low-fat and lean proteins, it becomes a healthy choice, but that's not all. You will cut back your sodium intake as well. A standard diet plan in this category allows you to have only 2300 mg of sodium on a daily basis; however, you can reduce your salt content to as low as 1500 mg salt per day.

Generally, a person consumes about 3400 mg of salt on a daily basis, which is why the reduction to 2000 or 1500 mg becomes an impressive choice for people. Reducing the sodium intake in your diet saves you from hypertension conditions.

At the core, the DASH diet includes low sodium food

choices only. You start using sodium-free ingredients and spices in your food. Ingredients like pasta or rice become salt-free. In fact, you are recommended to check every canned food item for the sodium content before buying.

The DASH Diet and Exercise

For this diet plan to work faster, you can enhance it with certain exercises. As you are reducing your calorie intake, it would be wise to burn calories at the same time to reach your weight loss goals faster.

When combined with cycling, walking, swimming, running and other exercises, this diet plan mimics a weight loss program; hence, you get to lose weight and control your high blood pressure at the same time. Apart from daily activities, a person should have at least 30 minutes of moderate level workout.

All in all, the DASH diet removes the high blood pressure triggers from your food. Also, you get to lose weight with calorie control and moderate exercise.

CHAPTER 2 – Develop Your Own DASH Diet Solution

Getting your own DASH diet solution is better to smoothly shift your meals. You don't have to force everything on yourself at once. A gradual shift toward a DASH diet provides more long-term sustainability. Many people start their diet with full force, but find it difficult to keep following, so they go back to their old food habits.

The first step should be to understand your own diet patterns. Find out the number of calories and type of nutrition you are consuming on a daily basis.

Let's discuss this in detail!

Steps to Start

A successful adoption of a DASH diet plan requires some simple steps in the beginning:

1. Prepare Your Diet Diary

You have multiple meals and snacks every day. Now,

it is time to keep a diary of what you are eating. Include a daily entry of your meals with the food items, the quantity of food items, and the time when you had the food. Similarly, include all the snacks that you eat in a day. This includes sugary beverages, chips, and other snacks you prefer at different times of your day.

After a few weeks, you will become aware of an overall calorie and nutritional value of your food habits. This will help you set a target for yourself.

2. Start Switching Snacks with Fruit

As mentioned before, it is difficult to suddenly switch your diet, so a gradual move would be a wise choice for you. Start by saving yourself from harmful snacks such as chips, sugary beverages, soda, and others. Whenever you feel like having a snack, choose a fruit salad, or have a glass of fruit juice. This is a great start to switching your diet.

3. Add at Least Two Vegetables in Your Daily Diet

The next step is including vegetables in your diet. Choose two green vegetables, and include them in your daily diet. You can even choose a combination of multiple vegetables for daily versatility. After the selection, make sure that you have one vegetable during your lunch and another vegetable at dinner.

This way, your meals will get the initial touch of the DASH diet.

4. Control Your Meat Food Content

People lose control of their weight and blood pressure due to a consistent meat intake in their diet, so the next step for you should be to balance your meat content. This process has two parts:

One, you need to switch to lean meat choices.

Second, you need to stop treating meats as the whole meal.

The second part is a little tricky. You need to start looking at meats as one portion of an overall meal, which is why there should be other portions, such as vegetables, beans, wheat pasta, and brown rice. In fact, it would be more effective if you choose one meat-free diet day every week.

5. Start Reading Nutritional Facts of Packaged Food Items

With a basic diet shift, you can now start pushing your diet towards DASH, but for that, you will require a knowledge of nutritional facts.

When buying packaged food items, look for products that have low saturated fats. Similarly, you need to know the cholesterol, sugar, sodium, transfat, and overall calories of foods you purchase.

6. Reduce Sodium in Your Diet

A big part of the DASH diet is controlling your sodium intake; however, you can't go too low on sodium either. The correct amount is about 1500 to 2300 mg on a daily basis, but it is most likely that you are taking in about 3400 mg of sodium every day.

So, start by ensuring that your canned fruits, vegetables, grains and other food items are low in sodium. There are low-sodium food products available on the market. Along with that, you should reduce the sodium, or salt, tolerance level in your taste. Start reducing the salt content in your meals by 1 teaspoon every day. One teaspoon usually measures to 2300 mg. You need to use this amount of sodium sparingly on a daily basis.

With these steps followed, you can prepare your own DASH diet solution, and gradually shift to a healthy lifestyle.

CHAPTER 3 – DASH DIET Nutrition

To prepare your own DASH diet solution, you also need to know the nutritional aspects of foods. There are certain food items you need to avoid, while others are beneficial in a DASH diet.

What Can You Eat?

1. Low-Fat Dairy Products:

Low-fat dairy products are permitted on this diet. You can make smoothies and shakes using low-fat milk and fruits such as strawberries, bananas and others.

Change your daily butter content with ricotta cheese. For instance, if you have a piece of toast made of whole grain, top it with low-fat cheese instead of butter.

Low-fat yogurt is also a good addition to your diet. You can have Greek yogurt as a mid-day snack, or use it in making your fruit salad, but make sure that the yogurt is plain and low in fat.

You can have two to three servings of low-fat dairy every day. For example, you can choose one cup of yogurt or one cup of milk in your diet per day.

2. Whole Grains:

Whole grains also come under the DASH diet. This category includes food items such as bread made of whole grain, brown rice, cereals made of whole grain, quinoa, bulgur and oatmeal.

You can have up to seven or eight servings of whole grains in your daily diet. For instance, one ounce of cereal, one slice of bread, or one half cup of brown rice is one serving. You can have one of any serving seven to eight times every day.

3. Fruits:

On the DASH diet, you are also required to include fruits--a lot of them. Choices such as pears, apples, berries and peaches are nutritious in the DASH diet. You can also include tropical fruit choices such as mango, pineapple and others.

Include dried, fresh, canned fruits and fruit juices in your diet. Just make sure that the canned ones are low in fat and sodium.

In one day, you can have four to five servings of fruits. Each serving can include one fruit or one half cup full of canned fruit or one half cup full of your favorite fruit juice.

4. Vegetables:

The DASH diet allows all kinds of vegetables such as carrots, broccoli, green beans, cauliflower, cabbage and others.

You are expected to add about four to five servings of vegetables in your diet. One serving can mean one cup of green veggies, one half cup of carrots, broccoli, tomatoes or squash or one half cup of vegetable juice such as carrots and spinach.

5. Lean Meat:

You are allowed to have meat, chicken or fish, but they have to be lean cuts. The servings should not exceed six and you should try to have meat-free days every week.

One serving of meat can include one egg or one ounce of cooked chicken, fish or meat.

6. Seeds and Nuts:

Almonds, hazelnuts, peanuts, sunflower seeds, walnuts, kidney seeds, flax seed, split peas and lentils all come under this category.

Seeds and nuts can come as four to five servings in a WEEK. In one serving, you can choose two tbsp. of seeds or nut butter, one half cup of cooked legumes or similar quantities of other seeds and nuts.

7. Vegetable Oil:

In a DASH diet, you are supposed to switch to vegetable oils. This includes corn oil, olive oil, canola oil, sunflower oil and other vegetable oils.

You can include two to three servings of vegetable oils in your daily diet.

What Food Should You Avoid?

Food items with high sugar, fat and salt content are avoided in the DASH diet. Some of those food items include:

- Cookies

- Too much alcohol

- Too much coffee

- Candy

- Salted nuts

- Chips

- Sugary beverages

- Soda

- Red meat

- Pizza

- High sodium packaged rice or pasta dishes

- Strong salad dressings

- High-fat dairy products

- Cured and cold cut meat

And much more!

CHAPTER 4 - High Carb vs Low Carb

In order to leverage the DASH diet as a weight loss program, you should understand the concept of high carbs and low carbs.

Carbohydrates have two major types--simple carbs and complex carbs.

Simple carbs include a high sugar content, and they get easily digested in the body cells. As a result, the blood sugar level increases faster with simple carbs, which impacts the blood pressure. Simple carbs are contained in candies, cakes, jam, chocolates, honey, in several fruits and in milk as well.

On the other hand, complex carbs become difficult to digest. The body cells gradually break down such carbs, and as a result, they become a steady source of energy. Such complex carbs are contained in nuts, root vegetables, whole grain and other sources.

In order to lose weight, you need to cut down your carb intake, and choose more complex carbs in your diet. Low carbs mean you take lesser calories on a daily basis, which results in a calorie deficiency in your body. This automatically starts reducing the weight in your body.

Hence, in order to understand the calorie quantity of high carb versus low carb, you need to evaluate your daily activities and daily energy requirements, and then you can decide how few carbs are enough to lose weight.

CHAPTER 5 - Weight Loss

The DASH Diet plan is more focused toward reducing blood pressure; however, the plan creates a nutritional system in your body, which helps in reducing weight as well. This is also true because of the impact of excess body weight on blood pressure. People with too much body weight tend to face high blood pressure problems; hence, experts suggest losing weight in order to control the blood pressure level in your body.

Can You Slim Down on the DASH Diet?

The DASH diet is effective in losing weight, but it controls the nutritional aspect only. It is your responsibility to decrease your daily calorie intake in order to lose weight. Also, it is advised to leverage moderate exercises to make the DASH diet more effective for weight loss.

Exercise Plan

Physical activities make the DASH diet more effective in terms of weight loss goals. People following this diet plan should have a parallel exercise plan as well.

A moderate exercise session of 30 minutes per day is enough, but you have to follow this plan consistently so choose an activity that you like the most.

Here is a sample exercise plan for you:

- Walk for at least 15 minutes.

- Run for 10 minutes at a moderate speed.

- Cycle for about 6 minutes.

- Spend 60 minutes doing household chores such as cleaning, laundry and others.

- Choose dance, swimming or any other activity and devote 15 minutes every day.

You can choose a combination of all exercises, or pick just one activity for a day.

The DASH Diet for Vegetarians

Vegetarians get unlimited food options in a DASH diet plan. If you are a vegetarian, focus on going additive-free with natural food items. With that approach, you can follow a vegetarian DASH diet plan every day.

Here is a DASH diet plan for vegetarians:

Breakfast:

- Orange- 1 medium
- Wheat bagel (whole wheat) and peanut butter- 1 bagel and 2 tbsp of unsalted peanut butter
- Coffee- decaffeinated
- Milk- 1 cup, fat-free or low-fat

Lunch:

- Vegetable salad- green veggies (1 cup), leafy veggies (1 cup),
- Almonds- 1/3 cup
- Milk or yogurt- 1 cup, fat-free
- Cooked beans- 1 cup

Dinner:

- Brown rice and vegetables- ½ cup
- Baked cod- 4 ounces
- Berries- 1 cup
- Herbal tea

Snacks:

- Greek yogurt- 1 cup, low-fat

- Wafers- 4

- Fruit salad- 1 cup

This is a sample plan, so you can switch one food item with other relevant options. For instance, you can have a glass of juice instead of an orange, or pick an apple in the morning.

DASH Dieting Tips for Long-Term Success

1. Use Aromatic Ingredients for Flavoring

Losing the taste is the biggest concern people have when thinking about salt reduction, but you can actually tackle this problem with flavorful ingredients such as vegetables, fruits, spices and herbs.

Certain vegetables, such as garlic, onions and peppers, have aromatic flavors. Cooking your recipes with such vegetables brings out flavors that take the place of salt beautifully. This way, you can reduce the salt content without compromising the taste.

Similar benefits are possible with herbs, such as parsley, rosemary, cilantro and others. Spices, such as cinnamon, black pepper, and cumin, effectively reduce the requirement of salt in a dish.

This means that you can have a low-sodium diet for a long time with flavorful ingredients.

2. Become Calorie-Focused

To make the DASH diet successful in the long run, you have to become calorie-focused. Your daily diet has to be less than 2100 calories per day. You need to divide this calorie amount into several portions:

- Fat: 27% of the total calories

- Carbohydrates- 55% of the total calories

- Protein- 18% of the total calories

- Saturated fats- less than 6% of the total calories

- Fibers- 30 grams

- Cholesterol- 150 mg or lesser

With this approach, you will successfully find yourself losing weight and living a healthy lifestyle.

3. Control Your Sugar Intake

Candy and sugary beverages become the biggest hurdle in this diet. You have to put an end to too much sugar intake in your body. You can't have more than one tbsp of sugar in the whole week. A sugary soda fills your body with too much sugar, so the long-term success of your diet plan depends on your control over additive sugar intake.

4. Stop or Limit Alcohol Consumption

Alcohol consumption is associated with high blood pressure. It also stops you from sticking to your daily caloric plan. More than three alcoholic drinks in a single day are harmful to your body.

For DASH diet success, you need to avoid, or at least control, your alcohol consumption and keep it to a minimum when possible.

Four-Week Meal Plan

You have already read the type of foods required for a DASH diet plan. Now, it is time to use those food items in your daily diet.

Diet Plan for 2000 Calories per Day

- Fruits: 4 to 5 servings

- Vegetables: 4 to 5 servings

- Grains: 7 to 8 servings

- Lean meat, poultry, or fish: less than 2 servings

- Low-fat dairy: 2 or 3 servings

- Sweets and fats: as limited as possible

- Nuts, legumes and seeds: 4 to 5 servings per week

Diet Plan for 2100 to 3100 Calories per Day

- Fruits: 4 to 6 servings

- Vegetables: 4 to 6 servings

- Grains: 6 to 12 servings

- Lean meat, poultry, or fish: 1½ to 2½ servings

- Low-fat dairy: 2 to 4 servings

- Sweets and fats: 2 to 4 servings

- Nuts, legumes and seeds: 4 to 6 servings per week

Everyday Meals to Be Followed for Four Weeks

For four weeks, you need to divide your daily food intake for the following meals:

- Breakfast

- Mid-morning snack

- Lunch

- Mid-afternoon snack

- Dinner

- Late-evening snack

Follow the following breakfast, lunch and dinner recipes for four weeks to reduce your waistline to the desired measurement.

CHAPTER 6 – Recipes for the DASH Diet Meal Plan

Breakfast Meal Recipes for a DASH Diet

Pineapple, Chickpea and Milk Smoothie

Number of Servings: 2

Ingredients

- Pineapple chunks- ¾ cup

- Milk- ¾ cup

- Chickpeas- ¾ cup, rinse and drain

- Ice- ½ cup

- Dates- 2 pitted

- Almond butter- 2 tbsp, no salt

- Turmeric- 2 tsp, ground

Steps to Cook

1. Mix every ingredient in a blender.

2. Blend to get a smooth texture.

3. You will get two glasses of smoothie.

Nutritional Information (per serving)

- Calories- 461

- Fat- 20 g

- Saturated fat- 9 g

- Sodium- 301 mg

- Cholesterol- 37 mg

- Carbohydrate- 75 g

- Protein- 32 g

Tangy Spinach and Banana Bowl

Number of Servings: 1

Ingredients

- Baby spinach - 1 cup, packed

- Orange juice- 1 cup

- Banana- 1

- Ice cubes- ½ cup

- Avocado- ½

- Pineapple- diced

- Flaxseeds- ground

Steps to Cook

1. Place banana, spinach, ice, avocado and orange juice in a blender.

2. Prepare a smooth texture by blending again and again.

3. Top with pineapple pieces, flaxseeds and blueberries.

4. You will get one breakfast serving.

Nutritional Information (per serving)

- Calories- 419

- Fat- 9 g

- Saturated fat- 0 g

- Sodium- 450 mg

- Cholesterol- 48 mg

- Carbohydrate- 45 g

- Protein- 9 g

Almond, Banana and Raspberries Smoothie

Number of Servings: 1

Ingredients

- Ripe banana- ½, medium sized

- Milk- ¼ cup, low-fat

- Frozen raspberries- 1 cup

- Almond butter- 1 tbsp

- Crushed ice- ½ cup

Steps to Cook

1. Cut banana into pieces and mix with other ingredients in a blender.

2. Blend until you get the desired smoothie texture.

3. You will have 1 serving for a perfect breakfast.

Nutritional Information (per serving)

- Calories- 238

- Fat- 15 g

- Saturated fat- 8 g

- Sodium- 301 mg

- Cholesterol- 47 mg

- Carbohydrate- 75 g

- Protein- 30 g

Ricotta and Pomegranate Grain Toast with Avocado

Number of Servings: 1

Ingredients
- Avocado - ½

- Bread - 1 slice, choose whole grain bread

- Pomegranate seeds- for topping

- Ricotta- 1 tsp

- Honey- just a little

Steps to Cook
1. In your toaster, prepare the bread slice. You can also toast it in your oven.

2. Place avocado pieces on the slice of toast.

3. Spread ricotta over the avocado pieces.

4. Pour a tiny amount of honey over, and sprinkle some pomegranate.

5. You will get one delicious serving of toast for breakfast.

Nutritional Information (per serving)

- Calories- 325

- Fat- 6 g

- Saturated fat- 1 g

- Sodium- 2 mg

- Cholesterol- 0 mg

- Carbohydrate- 30 g

- Protein- 3 g

Egg Parmesan Avocados

Number of Servings: 4

Ingredients

- Avocados- 2, ripe

- Pepper- ¼ tsp

- Coarse salt- ¼ tsp

- Eggs- 4 medium

- Olive oil- ½ tsp

- Parmesan- 1 tbsp, grated

- Herbs, paprika and diced tomatoes (for topping)

Steps to Cook

1. Prepare your oven by heating it to a temperature of 375 degrees F.

2. Cut avocados in four halves, and make a slice cut on the curvy sides of each piece so that the avocado sits still.

3. Use a scooper to remove the flesh of the avocado.

4. Place the avocado shells on a baking sheet. Sprinkle some salt and pepper, and brush with olive oil.

5. In each avocado cavity, pour 1 egg.

6. Top with cheese and cover with foil to bake in the preheated oven.

7. Allow 22 to 25 minutes for baking. The eggs should get settled properly.

8. Top with diced tomatoes, paprika and other toppings.

9. You will have 4 great servings with this recipe.

Nutritional Information (per serving)

- Calories- 220

- Fat- 5 g

- Saturated fat- 1 g

- Sodium- 151 mg

- Cholesterol- 13 mg

- Carbohydrate- 28 g

- Protein- 25 g

Apple and Cinnamon Oatmeal

Number of Servings: 4

Ingredients
- Apple- 3, large, small pieces

- Oats- 1 cup, steel-cut

- Cinnamon- 1 pinch, ground

- Peanut butter- 1 swirl

- Salt- 1 pinch

- Water- 4 cups

Steps to Cook
1. Cook your oats according to the directions offered on the package.

2. Cut apples into small-sized pieces and mix in the cooked oats.

3. Stir and add peanut butter. Mix properly for a smooth consistency.

4. Sprinkle 1 pinch of cinnamon on the top and

serve.

5. You will get 4 servings at once.

Nutritional Information (per serving)

- Calories- 453

- Fat- 4 g

- Saturated fat- 0 g

- Sodium- 89 mg

- Cholesterol- 4 mg

- Carbohydrate- 30 g

- Protein- 12 g

Tofu Cooked with Pepper Spinach and Mushrooms

Number of Servings: 2

Ingredients

- Olive oil- 1 tbsp, choose the extra-virgin version

- Tofu- 8 ounce, extra-firm, drained

- Bell pepper- 1, chopped

- Red onion- 1/4, chopped

- Button mushrooms- ½ cup, cut into slices

- Spinach- 2 cups, freshly chopped

- Garlic powder- 1 tsp

- Pepper and salt- ½ tsp

- Turmeric- ½ tbsp

- Nutritional yeast- ¼ cup

Steps to Cook

1. Properly remove the excess water from the tofu with a gentle squeeze.

2. Crumble the tofu in a large bowl.

3. Take a large skillet, put it over the heat with olive oil, include pepper and salt and let it heat for at least 4 to 5 minutes. Add the onions and the bell pepper. Make sure that the vegetables are soft. Add the mushrooms, and give another 3 minutes of cooking.

4. After cooking the vegetables, mix crumbled tofu in the same skillet, and mix with the vegetables. Cook this mixture for about 2 to 3 minutes, stirring occasionally.

5. Mix the nutritional yeast, turmeric and garlic, and include more pepper if required. Cook for 4 to 7 minutes, stirring occasionally, until you get a brown-colored tofu.

6. Finally, include the spinach, top the skillet with a lid and steam for about 3 minutes and serve.

7. You will get 2 servings.

Nutritional Information (per serving)

- Calories- 158

- Fat- 1 g

- Saturated fat- 0.2 g

- Sodium- 50 mg

- Cholesterol- 0 mg

- Carbohydrate- 13 g

- Protein- 5 g

Whole Grain Blueberry Pancakes

Number of Servings: 4

Ingredients

- Sorghum flour- ½ cup

- Oat flour- 1 cup

- Tapioca starch- 1/3 cup and more

- Teff flour- 2 tbsp

- Salt- ½ tsp

- Baking powder- 1 tbsp

- Flax meal- ½ tsp

- Sugar- 3½ tsp

- Cottage cheese- 1/3 cup

- Buttermilk- ¾ cup

- Vanilla extract- ½ tsp

- Eggs- 3

- Blueberries- 1 pint

- Canola oil- 4 tsp

- Water- 3 tbsp

- Maple syrup- ½ cup

- Salt- 1 pinch

- Lemon juice- 1 tsp

Steps to Cook

1. Take a large mixing bowl and mix all the dry flour ingredients.

2. Now, include all the wet ingredients in another bowl and mix properly.

3. Slowly pour the prepared wet mixture into the

dry one. Mix in batches to avoid lumps in the mixture.

4. Prepare a batter with a smooth consistency by whisking the mixture, and leave it to rest for about 12 to 15 minutes.

5. Prepare your griddle by preheating.

6. During this time, you can mix water, maple syrup, blueberries, lemon juice as well as salt. Make a warm compote by mixing these ingredients in a pot over medium heat and set aside.

7. Put some oil in the griddle and pour a small amount of batter on it to prepare your pancakes.

8. Cook until you get dry edges and bubbles on the top surface of the pancakes. It will take no more than 2 to 3 minutes.

9. Flip and give another 2 minutes on the other side of the pancake.

10. Do this with all the batter to prepare all of the pancakes.

11. You can serve it with a blueberry compote. Serves 4 people.

Nutritional Information (per serving)

- Calories- 511

- Fat- 2 g

- Saturated fat- 0.5 g

- Sodium- 115 mg

- Cholesterol- 0 mg

- Carbohydrate- 15 g

- Protein- 4 g

Fruit and Walnut Oatmeal

Number of Servings: 1

Ingredients
- Milk- 3 tbsp, fat-free

- Oats- 1/3, old-fashioned

- Honey- 1 tbsp

- Reduced-fat yogurt- 3 tbsp, plain

- Walnuts- 2 tbsp, toasted and chopped

- Fresh fruits- ½ cup

Steps to Cook
1. Take a sealable small-sized container and mix in the oats with the honey, yogurt and milk.

2. Place your favorite fruits and nuts on top.

3. Seal the container and refrigerate for about 30 to 50 minutes.

4. This recipe will give you 1 serving.

Nutritional Information (per serving)

- Calories- 345

- Fat- 13 g

- Saturated fat- 2 g

- Sodium- 53 mg

- Cholesterol- 4 mg

- Carbohydrate- 53 g

- Protein- 10 g

Tangy Chili Pineapple

Number of Servings: 6

Ingredients

- Brown sugar- 3 tbsp

- Pineapple- 1 fresh, cut into pieces

- Olive oil- 1 tbsp

- Lime juice- 1 tbsp

- Honey- 1 tbsp

- Salt- 1 dash

- Chili powder- 1½ tsp

Steps to Cook

1. Peel and cut pineapple lengthwise. Make sure you remove the eyes.

2. Mix all the other ingredients in a large bowl.

3. Use a soft brush to spread half of the prepared mixture all over the pineapple pieces.

4. Keep the rest of the mixture reserved.

5. Keep the heat on medium, and grill the pineapple pieces for about 3 to 4 minutes in a covered skillet to get a light brown color, and use the rest of the mixture for basting.

6. This great DASH diet breakfast recipe serves 6 people.

Nutritional Information (per serving)

- Calories- 97

- Fat- 2 g

- Saturated fat- 0 g

- Sodium- 4 mg

- Cholesterol- 0 mg

- Carbohydrate- 20 g

- Protein- 1 g

Dijon Tangy Shrimp Greens Salad

Number of Servings: 4

Ingredients

For Salad:

- Frozen corn- 1 cup

- Canola oil- 4 tsp, divided

- Salt- ¼ tsp

- Shrimp- 1 pound, devein and peel

- Salad greens- 8 cups, roughly torn

- Lemon and pepper- ½ tsp

- Nectarines- 2, small pieces

- Red onion- ½ cup, chopped pieces

- Grape tomatoes- 1 cup, halved

Other ingredients:

- Cider vinegar- 3 tbsp

- Orange juice- 1/3 cup

- Tarragon- 1 tbsp, freshly minced

- Dijon mustard- 1 ½ tsp

- Honey- 1 tsp

Steps to Cook

1. Take a small-sized bowl and mix vinegar, orange juice, honey and mustard. Mix properly, then include tarragon as well.

2. Using a large skillet, heat some oil. Include corn and cook for about 1 to 3 minutes, stirring. Set aside.

3. Use lemon pepper along with salt to season the shrimp. Use the previously used skillet with more oil to cook shrimp over medium heat. This should take about 4 to 5 minutes. Shrimp will become pink and opaque. Mix this with the cooked corn.

4. Use a large bowl to mix all the other ingredients with the mixture of shrimp and corn.

5. Makes 4 servings.

Nutritional Information (per serving)

- Calories- 252

- Fat- 7 g

- Saturated fat- 1 g

- Sodium- 448 mg

- Cholesterol- 38 mg

- Carbohydrate- 27 g

- Protein- 23 g

Brown Rice, Mango and Vanilla Pudding

Number of Servings: 1

Ingredients
- Brown rice- 1 cup, long grain, uncooked

- Salt- ¼ tsp

- Water- 2 cups

- Soy milk- 1 cup, vanilla flavored

- Ripe mango- 1 medium

- Ground cinnamon- ½ tsp

- Sugar- 2 tbsp

- Mango pieces for topping

- Vanilla extract- 1 tsp

Steps to Cook
1. In a saucepan, include the salt and water and boil, then add the rice in the boiling salt water.

2. Reduce the temperature, and simmer with a

covered lid for about 30 to 40 minutes. Make sure that the rice is tender.

3. During this time, prepare a mash of mango pieces using a fork.

4. Add the mashed mango, cinnamon, milk and sugar to the rice. Remove the cover and cook for about 12 to 15 minutes. Stir from time to time to check the consistency.

5. Move away from heat, and add the vanilla extract into the hot pudding.

6. Let it rest until it reaches room temperature, and then refrigerate overnight.

7. Use chopped mango as a topping when serving in the morning.

Nutritional Information (per serving)

- Calories- 275

- Fat- 3 g

- Saturated fat- 0 g

- Sodium- 176 mg

- Cholesterol- 0 mg

- Carbohydrate- 58 g

- Protein- 6 g

Cheese and Asparagus Tortilla Omelet

Number of Servings: 1

Ingredients

- Milk- 1 tbsp, fat-free

- Egg whites- 2, large

- Egg- 1

- Pepper- 1/8 tsp

- Parmesan cheese- 2 tsp, grated

- Butter- 1 tsp, low-sodium, low-fat

- Asparagus- 4, freshly sliced

- Green onion- 1, chopped

- Tortilla- 1 wrap, whole wheat

Steps to Cook

1. In a large bowl, mix together the milk, egg, cheese, egg whites and pepper.

2. Warm a skillet over heat using cooking spray. Include the asparagus and cook for about 2 to 4 minutes, stirring occasionally. Place the cooked asparagus into a dish or bowl.

3. In the same heated skillet, add the butter, and pour the mixture of egg and cheese on to it.

Cook properly making sure the sides of the omelet are thoroughly cooked.

4. Top half of the side of the omelet with the cooked asparagus and chopped onions, and then fold the other half portion over it.

5. Remove and wrap in the tortilla.

Nutritional Information (per serving)

- Calories- 319

- Fat- 13 g

- Saturated fat- 5 g

- Sodium- 444 mg

- Cholesterol- 25 mg

- Carbohydrate- 28 g

- Protein- 21 g

Lunch Meal Recipes for a DASH Diet

Dijon Mustard Shrimp with a Corn Green Salad

Number of Servings: 4

Ingredients

- Cider vinegar- 3 tbsp

- Orange juice- 1/3 cup

- Tarragon- 1 tbsp, freshly minced

- Honey- 1 ½ tsp

- Frozen corn- 1 cup

- Canola oil- 4 tsp, divided

- Pepper and lemon seasoning- ½ tsp

- Shrimp- 1 pound, peel and devein

- Salad greens- 8 cups, mixed and torn

- Salt- ¼ tsp

- Nectarines- 2, pieces cut

- Red onion- ½ cup, chopped

- Grape tomatoes- 1 cup, cut in halves

Steps to Cook

1. In a medium-sized bowl, mix the vinegar, orange juice, honey and mustard. Whisk properly, and include tarragon.

2. Choose an appropriate sized skillet and heat the oil, keeping the heat medium-high. Include the corn, and cook to get a crispy and tender texture, stirring occasionally. This should take about 2 minutes.

3. Season and salt the shrimp. Use the previously-used skillet with more heated oil to cook the shrimp. In 4 to 5 minutes of cooking, you will see the pink color of the shrimp, and then add the corn, stirring occasionally.

4. In a large bowl, mix the cooked mixture with all the other ingredients.

5. Serves 4.

Nutritional Information (per serving)

- Calories- 252

- Fat- 7 g

- Saturated fat- 1 g

- Sodium- 448 mg

- Cholesterol- 38 mg

- Carbohydrate- 27 g

- Protein- 23 g

Tomato and Chili Pork Chops

Number of Servings: 6

Ingredients

- Pork loin- 6 chops, lean meat, boneless

- Butter- 4 tsp, divided, low-fat, unsalted

- Apples- 3, sliced

- Onion- 1, chopped

- Sugar- 4 tsp

- Tomatoes- 1 can of 28 ounces

- Salt- ½ tsp

- Curry powder- 2 tsp

- Brown rice- 4 cups, cooked

- Chili powder- ½ tsp

- Toasted almonds- 2 tbsp

Steps to Cook

1. Use a stockpot and include 2 tsp of butter and heat, keeping the heat medium-high. Divide the pork chops into various batches, and brown them in the heated butter.

2. Use the same pot to cook the onion in more butter, stirring. Cook the onions for 3 minutes, and then add the tomatoes, apples, curry powder, sugar, chili powder and salt. Boil, and then reduce to a simmer, breaking the tomato pieces.

3. Now, add the browned pork pieces, and let it simmer for another 4 to 5 minutes. After the first 3 minutes, make sure you turn the pork pieces.

4. Use a thermometer to check that the internal temperature is about 145 degrees.

5. Serve with cooked rice and roasted almonds. You will get 6 servings with this recipe.

Nutritional Information (per serving)

- Calories- 478

- Fat- 14 g

- Saturated fat- 5 g

- Sodium- 475 mg

- Cholesterol- 39 mg

- Carbohydrate- 50 g

- Protein- 38 g

Whole Wheat Pasta with Cooked Chicken and Veggies

Number of Servings: 6

Ingredients

- Canola oil- 2 tsp

- Pasta- 6 ounces, whole wheat

- Julienned carrots- 2 cups

- Snap peas- 10 ounces, trimmed and strip cuts

- Peanut sauce- 1 cup

- Cooked chicken- 2 cups, shredded

- Cilantro- chopped

- Cucumber- 1, lengthwise cut, seeded and sliced

Steps to Cook

1. Cook the pasta according to the directions provided on the package. Drain properly.

2. Then, choose a large skillet, and heat the available oil, keeping the heat medium-high.

3. Add the carrots and snap peas, and cook for about 7 to 8 minutes, stirring. Add the peanut sauce over the pasta, and place it in the skillet as well. Then, add the shredded chicken.

4. Combine, stir and toss properly.

5. Use cucumber and cilantro as toppings before serving. You will get 6 servings.

Nutritional Information (per serving)

- Calories- 403

- Fat- 15 g

- Saturated fat- 3 g

- Sodium- 432 mg

- Cholesterol- 42 mg

- Carbohydrate- 43 g

- Protein- 25 g

Tomato and Basil Soup with Carrots and Green Beans

Number of Servings: 9

Ingredients

- Carrots- 1 cup, roughly chopped

- Onion- 1 cup, finely chopped

- Vegetable broth- 6 cups, low-sodium

- Butter- 2 tsp

- Garlic- 1 clove, freshly minced

- Green beans- 1 pound, into pieces

- Basil- ¼ cup, freshly minced

- Tomatoes- 3 cup, freshly diced

- Pepper- ¼ tsp

- Salt- ½ tsp

Steps to Cook

1. In a large saucepan, sautéing the carrots and onions in heated butter. This should take about 4 to 5 minutes.

2. Stir in the garlic, and heat another minute to get the fragrance of the garlic, then add the broth and beans and boil the whole mixture.

3. Now, decrease the heat and simmer with the lid covered for about 15 to 20 minutes. Make sure all the veggies become tender.

4. Lastly, add the tomatoes, pepper and salt. Give another 5 minutes to simmer and serve warm.

5. You will get up to 9 servings with this.

Nutritional Information (per serving)

- Calories- 58

- Fat- 1 g

- Saturated fat- 1 g

- Sodium- 535 mg

- Cholesterol- 2 mg

- Carbohydrate- 10 g

- Protein- 4 g

Paprika and Mushroom Sole with Tomato and Green Onions

Number of Servings: 4

Ingredients

- Mushrooms- 2 cups, freshly sliced

- Butter- 2 tbsp

- Sole- 4 fillets, wild-caught, each fillet with 4 ounces

- Garlic- 2 cloves, freshly minced

- Pepper and lemon seasoning- ¼ tsp

- Paprika- ¼ tsp

- Tomato- 1, medium-sized, chopped

- Cayenne pepper- 1/8 tsp

- Green onions- 2, slices

Steps to Cook

1. In a large pan, add butter to warm, keeping the heat medium-high. Add the mushrooms and cook for about 3 minutes to make it tender, stirring. Now, you can add the garlic into the mixture and cook about 1 more minute.

2. Shift the fillets to the pan, and season with pepper and lemon seasoning, paprika and cayenne.

3. Cover the top with the lid, and cook for about 6 to 10 minutes, keeping the heat medium.

4. Use a fork to check the flaking of the fish.

5. Add the green onions and tomato before serving.

6. You will get 4 servings.

Nutritional Information (per serving)

- Calories- 174

- Fat- 7 g

- Saturated fat- 4 g

- Sodium- 166 mg

- Cholesterol- 49 mg

- Carbohydrate- 4 g

- Protein- 23 g

Beef, Walnuts and Spinach with Cheesy Penne

Number of Servings: 4

Ingredients

- Beef tenderloin- 2 steaks, lean mcat, with each steak being 6 ounces

- Penne pasta- 2 cups, whole wheat, uncooked

- Pepper- ¼ tsp

- Salt- ¼ tsp

- Grape tomatoes- 2 cups, cut into halves

- Walnuts- ¼ cup, finely chopped

- Pesto- 1/3 cup

- Gorgonzola cheese- ¼ cup, low-fat

Steps to Cook

1. Follow the package directions to cook the penne pasta.

2. Use pepper and salt to season the lean steaks. Keep the heat medium, and grill for about 6 minutes on each side.

3. Drain the cooked pasta, and move it to a large bowl for mixing.

4. Add the tomatoes, spinach, walnuts and pesto

in the pasta and mix properly. Then, make slices of the steak and transfer it to the pasta mixture as well.

5. Top with cheese before serving. You will get 4 servings.

Nutritional Information (per serving)

- Calories- 532

- Fat- 22 g

- Saturated fat- 6 g

- Sodium- 434 mg

- Cholesterol- 40 mg

- Carbohydrate- 49 g

- Protein- 35 g

Zucchini Beans Quinoa

Number of Servings: 4

Ingredients

- Quinoa- 1 cup, rinsed and properly drained

- Olive oil- 1 tbsp

- Zucchini- 1 medium, chopped

- Garbanzo beans- ¾ cup, rinsed and properly

drained

- Water- 2 cups

- Feta cheese- ½ cup

- Tomato- 1, finely chopped

- Greek olives- ¼ cup, properly chopped

- Pepper- ¼ tsp

- Basil- 2 tbsp, freshly minced

Steps to Cook

1. In a large saucepan, heat oil, keeping the heat medium-high.

2. Add the garlic and quinoa, and cook for about 3 minutes until the quinoa is a light brown color, stirring occasionally.

3. Add water and zucchini, and bring this mixture to a boil, then decrease the heat to simmer. Keep the pan covered for simmering for about 14 to 15 minutes. This will allow all the liquid to be absorbed into the mixture.

4. Now, you can stir all the other ingredients and cook for about 2 extra minutes.

5. This will get you 4 servings.

Nutritional Information (per serving)

- Calories- 310

- Fat- 11 g

- Saturated fat- 3 g

- Sodium- 353 mg

- Cholesterol- 8 mg

- Carbohydrate- 42 g

- Protein- 11 g

Grapefruit Pork with Egg Noodles

Number of Servings: 8

Ingredients

- Dried oregano- 1 tsp

- Pork roast- 1, 4 pounds, lean sirloin

- Ground ginger- ½ tsp

- Onions- 2, thin wedges

- Pepper- ½ tsp

- Sugar- 1 tbsp

- Orange juice- 1 cup and more, divided

- Steak sauce- 1 tbsp

- Grapefruit juice- 1 tbsp

- Orange zest- 1 tsp, grated

- Soy sauce- 1 tbsp, low-sodium

- Cornstarch- 3 tbsp

- Salt- ½ tsp

- Oregano- freshly minced

- Egg noodles- cooked

Steps to Cook

1. Divide the pork pieces into two halves. Take a small-sized bowl and mix together pepper, ginger and oregano. Use this mixture to rub all over the pork pieces.

2. Take a non-stick pan large enough for the roast. Coat with some cooking spray, and cook the pork pieces on mild heat for browning.

3. Now, place the pork and onions into a slow cooker.

4. In a small bowl, mix the grapefruit juice, sugar, orange juice, soy sauce and steak sauce together. Pour this mixture into the cooker.

5. Set the heat to a low setting, and cover with a lid. Cook for about 5 hours.

6. Take out the onion and meat pieces and place in a bowl.

7. In the remaining mixture, add the cornstarch

and boil to get a thick consistency.

8. Add the salt and orange zest in the mixture of onion and meat.

9. Serve with cooked noodles in 8 serving plates.

Nutritional Information (per serving)

- Calories- 289

- Fat- 10 g

- Saturated fat- 4 g

- Sodium- 326 mg

- Cholesterol- 42 mg

- Carbohydrate- 13 g

- Protein- 35 g

Tangy Pineapple Tilapia

Number of Servings: 8

Ingredients

- Green onions- 2, chopped

- Pineapple- 2 cups, freshly cubed

- Cilantro- ¼ cup, freshly minced

- Green pepper- ¼ cup, properly chopped

- Salt- 1/8 + ¼ tsp, divided

- Lime juice- 4 tsp + 2 tbsp, divided

- Canola oil- 1 tbsp

- Cayenne pepper- just a dash

- Pepper- 1/8 tsp

- Tilapia- 8 fillets, about 4 ounces in one fillet

Steps to Cook

1. Use a small bowl to prepare the pineapple salsa. Mix the green onions, pineapple, cilantro, green pepper, and cayenne, 1/8 tsp of salt and about 4 tsp of lime juice. Mix and bag to refrigerate.

2. Now, drizzle a mixture of the lime juice and oil over the Tilapia fillets. Season with the rest of the salt and pepper.

3. Rub some cooking oil on the cooking rack for grilling.

4. Grill the fillets, covered with a lid for about 2 to 3 minutes, keeping the heat medium-high.

5. Use a fork to check the flakiness of the cooked fish.

6. Serve with the pineapple salsa. You can get 8 servings with this recipe.

Nutritional Information (per serving)

- Calories- 131

- Fat- 3 g

- Saturated fat- 1 g

- Sodium- 152 mg

- Cholesterol- 35 mg

- Carbohydrate- 6 g

- Protein- 21 g

Tuna and Pepper Kebab Sticks

Number of Servings: 4

Ingredients

- Green onions- 4, chopped

- Frozen corn- ½ cup, thawed

- Fresh parsley- 2 tbsp, chopped

- Jalapeno- 1, remove seeds and chop

- Tuna steaks- 1 pound, cubed

- Lime juice- 2 tbsp

- Ground pepper- 1 tsp

- Mango- 1, peeled and cubed

- Red peppers- 2, make large pieces

Steps to Cook

1. In a large bowl, mix the onions, corn, parsley, jalapeno and lime juice. Set aside.

2. Use pepper to coat the tuna fillets, and then make kebab sticks with red peppers, mango, and tuna.

3. Grease your grill rack, and carefully place all the kebab skewers. Keeping the heat on medium, cook until peppers are tender and tuna the tuna is pink.

4. Cooking about 9 to 12 minutes.

5. You will get about 4 servings.

Nutritional Information (per serving)

- Calories- 205

- Fat- 2 g

- Saturated fat- 0 g

- Sodium- 50 mg

- Cholesterol- 48 mg

- Carbohydrate- 20 g

- Protein- 29 g

Black Bean, Parsley and Pepper Frittata

Number of Servings: 6

Ingredients

- Egg whites- 3, large

- Salsa- ¼ cup

- Egg- 6, large

- Pepper- ¼ tsp

- Salt- ¼ tsp

- Olive oil- 1 tbsp

- Pepper- ¼ tsp

- Red bell pepper- 1/3 cup, properly chopped

- Green bell pepper- 1/3 cup, properly chopped

- Garlic- 2 cloves, minced

- Green onions- 3, chopped properly

- Cheddar cheese- ½ cup, shredded

- Black beans- 1 cup, rinse and drain

- Cilantro, olives, and salsa for toppings

Steps to Cook

1. In a large bowl, mix the salsa, egg whites,

parsley, eggs, salt and parsley.

2. Use an ovenproof pan, and heat the oil in it. Include the green onions and peppers and cook for about 4 to 5 minutes, stirring, until the peppers and onions are tender. Then, you can add the garlic and cook for one more minute.

3. Stir the beans into the same mixture, and reduce the heat to medium-low. Pour in the egg mixture. Cook without a lid for about 5 to 6 minutes, and then let the mixture settle.

4. Cut into wedges and serve with the available toppings. You will get 6 servings.

Nutritional Information (per serving)

- Calories- 183

- Fat- 10 g

- Saturated fat- 4 g

- Sodium- 378 mg

- Cholesterol- 19 mg

- Carbohydrate- 9 g

- Protein- 13 g

Turkey Breast and Spinach Soup

Number of Servings: 6

Ingredients

- Carrots- 5, chopped

- Canola oil- 1 tbsp

- Barley- 2/3 cup, immediate-cooking

- Onion- 1, chopped

- Turkey breast- 2 cups, cooked and cooked

- Chicken broth- 6 cups, low-sodium

- Pepper- ½ tsp

- Baby spinach- 2 cups, fresh

Steps to Cook

1. Pour oil into a large pan, and cook over medium heat. Add the onion and carrots, and cook for about 5 to 6 minutes, stirring. This will give the carrots a tender texture.

2. Add the broth and barley and let it boil for one minute, then decrease the heat and simmer for about 12 to 15 minutes, keeping the pan covered.

3. Mix the spinach, pepper and turkey pieces, and heat for consistency.

4. You will get 6 servings.

Nutritional Information (per serving)

- Calories- 208

- Fat- 4 g

- Saturated fat- 1 g

- Sodium- 662 mg

- Cholesterol- 37 mg

- Carbohydrate- 23 g

- Protein- 21 g

Chicken and Veggies Lettuce Cups

Number of Servings: 4

Ingredients

- Ground ginger- 1 tsp

- Chicken breasts- ¾ pound, cubed

- Pepper- ¼ tsp

- Salt- ¼ tsp

- Shredded carrots- 1½ cups

- Olive oil- 2 tsp

- Green onions- 4, chopped

- Sweet cherries- 1¼ cups

- Rice vinegar- 2 tbsp

- Almonds- 1/3 cup

- Teriyaki sauce- 2 tbsp

- Lettuce leaves- 8

- Honey- 1 tbsp

Steps to Cook

1. Use the pepper, salt and ginger to season the chicken.

2. Take out your non-stick skillet, and coat it with some cooking spray. Heat the oil in the skillet, keeping the heat medium-high. Add the seasoned chicken, and cook for about 4 to 5 minutes until golden brown.

3. After cooking, move the chicken away from the heat and mix the green onions, cherries, carrots and almonds.

4. In another bowl, mix together the teriyaki sauce, vinegar, and honey. Add the cooked chicken mixture in this too.

5. Fill the lettuce with this mixture, and create multiple cups.

6. You will get 4 servings.

Nutritional Information (per serving)

- Calories- 257

- Fat- 10 g

- Saturated fat- 1 g

- Sodium- 381 mg

- Cholesterol- 47 mg

- Carbohydrate- 22 g

- Protein- 21 g

Steak and Vegetable Pasta with Lime and Cilantro Dressing

Number of Servings: 4

Ingredients

- Beef steak- 1, top sirloin, lean protein (about ¾ pound)

- Ground cumin- ¼ tsp

- Salt- ¼ tsp

- Poblano peppers- 3, with the seeds removed and halved

- Pepper- ¼ tsp

- Sweetcorn- 2, and remove the husks

- Olive oil- 1 tbsp

- Sweet onion- 1, cut into rings

- Tomatoes- 2, large

- Whole grain pasta- 2 cups

For the dressing:

- Olive oil- 1 tbsp

- Lime juice- ¼ cup

- Ground cumin- ¼ tsp

- Salt- ¼ tsp

- Cilantro- 1/3 cup, freshly chopped

- pepper- ¼ tsp

Steps to Cook

1. Use the cumin, pepper and salt to coat the steak. Use a brush to oil the onion rings, corn and poblano peppers.

2. Use a medium heat to grill the coated steak for about 7 to 8 minutes in a covered dish. Make sure the internal temperature reaches about 140 to 150 degrees.

3. Now, for 9 to 10 minutes, grill the veggies while turning them occasionally.

4. Cook the pasta as directed in the package.

During this time, you can cut the tomatoes, onion and peppers. Also, cut the corn from the cob. Make a mixture of all these veggies in a large bowl.

5. In a different bowl, make your dressing with the oil, lime juice, salt, pepper and cumin. Stir the cilantro last.

6. Remove the water from the cooked pasta, and mix with all the vegetables. In the mixture, pour in the prepared dressing.

7. Finally, mix the sliced steak pieces in the pasta to serve.

8. You will get 4 servings.

Nutritional Information (per serving)

- Calories- 456

- Fat- 13 g

- Saturated fat- 3 g

- Sodium- 378 mg

- Cholesterol- 34 mg

- Carbohydrate- 58 g

- Protein- 30 g

Beef Soup with Potatoes, Carrots and Green Veggies

Number of Servings: 8

Ingredients

- Onion- 1, chopped

- Ground beef- 1½ pounds, pick 90% lean beef

- Julienned carrots- 10 ounces

- Garlic- 2 cloves, minced

- Tomato paste- ¼ cup

- Celery- 2 ribs, chopped

- Tomatoes- 1 can, diced, undrained

- Zucchini- 1, chopped

- Cabbage- 1½ cups, shred

- Green beans- ½ cup, frozen

- Red potato- 1, medium, finely chopped

- Dried oregano- ½ tsp

- Dried basil- 1 tsp

- Pepper- ¼ tsp

- Salt- ¼ tsp

- Beef broth- 4 cans, low-sodium

Steps to Cook

1. Use a stockpot, and add the garlic, onion and beef. Keeping the heat medium, cook this mixture for about 7 to 8 minutes. Add the celery and carrots to cook for another 7 to 8 minutes, stirring. Add the tomato paste and cook one more minute.

2. Add the cabbage, tomatoes, potato, zucchini, green beans, broth and seasonings. Let the mixture boil once, then simmer for about 30 to 40 minutes to get the desired consistency.

3. Serve warm.

4. You will get 8 servings with this recipe.

Nutritional Information (per serving)

- Calories- 207

- Fat- 7 g

- Saturated fat- 3 g

- Sodium- 621 mg

- Cholesterol- 27 mg

- Carbohydrate- 14 g

- Protein- 21 g

Green Chili Rice with Pinto Beans

Number of Servings: 4

Ingredients

- Corn- 1 cup

- Olive oil- 1 tbsp

- Garlic- 2 cloves, minced

- Onion- 1, chopped

- Ground cumin- 1½ tsp

- Chili powder- 1½ tsp

- Pinto beans- 15 ounce can, rinse and drain

- Green chilies- 4 ounce can, chopped

- Brown rice- 1 package, ready for serving

- Fresh cilantro- ¼ cup, chopped

- Salsa- ½ cup

- Cheddar cheese- ¼ cup, shredded

- Romaine- 1 bunch, quartered lengthwise

Steps to Cook

1. Take a large skillet and warm some oil, keeping the heat medium-high.

2. Include the onion and corn in the skillet and stir for about 4 to 5 minutes, stirring. When the onion gets tender, add the garlic, cumin and chili powder, and let the mixture cook for about 1 to 2 minutes.

3. Add the green chilies, beans, cilantro, salsa and rice. Heat and stir properly.

4. Use the romaine wedges when serving, and top with shredded cheese.

5. You will get 4 servings with this recipe.

Nutritional Information (per serving)

- Calories- 331

- Fat- 8 g

- Saturated fat- 2 g

- Sodium- 465 mg

- Cholesterol- 7 mg

- Carbohydrate- 50 g

- Protein- 12 g

Crispy Turkey with Tomato and Pepper Delight

Number of Servings: 6

Ingredients

- Sugar- ½ tsp

- Vinegar- 1 tbsp, a red wine version

- Olive oil- 2 tbsp

- Dried oregano- ¼ tsp

- Green pepper- 1, chopped

- Salt- ¼ tsp

- Red onion- ¼ cup

- Celery- 1 rib, chopped

- Tomatoes- 3, medium-sized

- Fresh basil- 1 tbsp, sliced

For the turkey:

- Lemon juice- 2 tbsp

- Egg- 1 large

- Parmesan cheese- ½ cup, shredded

- Breadcrumbs- 1 cup

- Pepper and lemon seasoning- 1 tsp

- Walnuts- ½ cup, chopped

- Salt- ¼ tsp

- Turkey breast- 20 ounces, tenderloins, lean protein

- Olive oil- 3 tbsp

- Pepper- ¼ tsp

- Fresh basil

Steps to Cook

1. Take a bowl and mix the vinegar, oil, oregano, sugar and salt. Include the celery, green pepper, basil, and onion in it. Cut large wedges of the tomato, and mix that in as well.

2. Use a shallow bowl to mix the lime juice with the egg.

3. In another similar bowl, you can combine the cheese with breadcrumbs, and add the pepper, lemon and walnuts.

4. Make slices of tenderloins, and use a mallet to flatten the cut slices. Season all the slices with salt and pepper.

5. Now you can dip every slice once into the egg mixture and once into the mixture of breadcrumbs. Pat and do this with every tenderloin slice.

6. Keeping the heat medium-high, you can heat some oil in a large skillet. Add 1/3 of the turkey slices to fry. This will take about 3 minutes on each side to become golden brown.

7. Serve with the chili and tomato mixture prepared earlier.

8. You will get 6 servings with this recipe.

Nutritional Information (per serving)

- Calories- 351

- Fat- 21 g

- Saturated fat- 3 g

- Sodium- 458 mg

- Cholesterol- 38 mg

- Carbohydrate- 13 g

- Protein- 29 g

Tangy Strawberry, Cheese and Beef Salad

Number of Servings: 4

Ingredients

- Salt- ½ tsp

- Beef steak- 1 pound, top sirloin

- Olive oil- 2 tsp

- Pepper- ¼ tsp

- Lime juice- 2 tbsp

For the salad:

- Strawberries- 2 cups, freshly halved

- Romaine- 1 bunch, cups torn

- Blue cheese- ¼ cup, low-fat, crumbled

- Red onion- ¼ cup, slices

- Balsamic vinaigrette- low-fat

- Walnuts- ¼ cup, toasted, chopped

Steps to Cook

1. Use the salt and pepper to season the beef steak.

2. Keeping the heat medium, warm some oil in a large skillet. Cook the seasoned steak for 6 to 7 minutes on each side. Set aside to rest for 4 to 8 minutes. Now, cut into strips and pour on the lime juice.

3. On a platter, combine the onion, strawberries and romaine. Top with walnuts and cheese.

4. Serve using vinaigrette.

5. You will get 4 servings with this recipe.

Nutritional Information (per serving)

- Calories- 289

- Fat- 15 g

- Saturated fat- 4 g

- Sodium- 425 mg

- Cholesterol- 12 mg

- Carbohydrate- 12 g

- Protein- 29 g

Chickpeas, Sweet Potatoes and Veggie Wraps

Number of Servings: 6

Ingredients

- Chickpeas- 2 cans of 15 ounces, and rinse and drain

- Sweet potatoes- 2, peel and cut into cubes

- Canola oil- 3 tbsp, divided

- Red onion- 1, chopped

- Salt- ½ tsp, divided

- Garam masala- 2 tsp

- Greek yogurt- 1 cup, choose a plain version

- Garlic- 2 cloves, minced

- Ground cumin- 1 tsp

- Lemon juice- 1 tbsp

- Baby spinach- 2 cups

- Cilantro- ¼ cup, freshly minced

- Wheat pita packets- 6, halved, warmed, and choose a whole wheat version

Steps to Cook

1. Preheat the oven to 400 degrees.

2. Put the potatoes in a bowl that is safe for microwave cooking. Cover the bowl, and microwave on high for 5 minutes.

3. Take out the potatoes and mix with onion and chickpeas. Add some oil along with the salt and garam masala.

4. In a large pan, spread the whole mixture. Roast for about 12 to 15 minutes to get tender potatoes.

5. Now, in another bowl for microwave cooking, put in the garlic and the rest of the oil. Brown the garlic in the microwave for 1 to 2 minutes. Stir in the lemon juice, yogurt, salt, and cumin.

6. Toss the cooked potato mixture, adding the

baby spinach.

7. Take 12 halves of the pitas, and fill them with the mixture and sauce, and top with cilantro.

8. Serves 6 people.

Nutritional Information (per serving)

- Calories- 462

- Fat- 15 g

- Saturated fat- 3 g

- Sodium- 662 mg

- Cholesterol- 10 mg

- Carbohydrate- 72 g

- Protein- 14 g

Creamy Asparagus and Thyme Soup

Number of Servings: 12

Ingredients

- Olive oil- 1 tbsp

- Butter- 1 tbsp

- Onion- 1, chopped

- Fresh asparagus- 2 pounds, trim and cut pieces

- Salt- ½ tsp

- Carrot- 1, thin slices

- Dried thyme- ¼ tsp

- Pepper- ¼ tsp

- Brown rice- 2/3 cup, long grain, uncooked

- Sour cream- low-fat

- Chicken broth- 6 cups, low-sodium

Steps to Cook

1. Use a large stockpot to heat the oil and butter, keeping the heat medium. Then, add the seasonings and vegetables. Cook this mixture about 9 to 10 minutes. Cook, stirring occasionally to get tender vegetables.

2. Add the chicken broth, as well as the rice. Bring this whole mixture to a boil, then reduce the heat, and let the mixture simmer for about 40 to 45 minutes keeping the pot covered. Stir from time to time and check the readiness of the rice.

3. Transfer the soup to a blender to make a puree-like consistency. You can do this in multiple batches.

4. Include the sour cream when serving.

5. You will get 12 servings.

Nutritional Information (per serving)

- Calories- 79

- Fat- 3 g

- Saturated fat- 1 g

- Sodium- 401 mg

- Cholesterol- 3 mg

- Carbohydrate- 11 g

- Protein- 4 g

Sweet Potato and Kale Rice

Number of Servings: 2

Ingredients

- Garlic salt- ¼ tsp

- Rice- ¾ cup, long grain, uncooked

- Olive oil- 3 tbsp, divided

- Water- 1½ cups

- Red onion- 1, finely chopped

- Sweet potato- 1, peel and dice

- Black beans- 15 ounces, rinse and drain

- Fresh kale- 4 cups, chopped

- Lime wedges

- Sweet and chili sauce- 2 tbsp

Steps to Cook

1. In a large saucepan, add the rice and fill the pot with water. Also add the garlic salt into the mixture. Boil, then simmer for about 16 to 20 minutes at reduced heat. Leave to rest for at least 10 minutes.

2. During this time, you can heat 2 tbsp of oil in a skillet, and sauté the sweet potato, keeping the heat medium-high. This should take about 5 to 8 minutes. Then, add the onion and cook for 5 minutes more, stirring. Put in the kale and cook for an additional 2 to 5 minutes, stirring. Add the beans and stir.

3. Now, you can put the chili sauce and the rest of the oil into the rice, then mix, and add the sweet potato mixture in as well and stir.

4. Place lime wedges on the side.

5. Serves 4 people.

Nutritional Information (per serving)

- Calories- 435

- Fat- 11 g

- Saturated fat- 2 g

- Sodium- 405 mg

- Cholesterol- 0 mg

- Carbohydrate- 74 g

- Protein- 10 g

Mahi Mahi Cardamom Tacos

Number of Servings: 6

Ingredients

- Ground cardamom- 1 tsp

- Olive oil- ¼ cup

- Salt- 1 tsp

- Paprika- 1 tsp

- Mahi-mahi- 6 fillets, each fillet should weigh about 6 ounces

- Pepper- 1 tsp

- Red cabbage- 2 cups, finely chopped

- Corn tortillas- 12

- Salsa verde

- Cilantro- 1 cup, freshly chopped

- Pepper sauce

- Lime wedges- 4

Steps to Cook

1. In a large baking dish, mix together the cardamom, olive oil, paprika, and pepper, as well as the salt. Place the mahi-mahi fillets into the mixture, and turnover for complete coating. Refrigerate the fillets for about 20 to 35 minutes.

2. After marinating the fillets, drain and get rid of the marinade. Oil a grill rack and place the fillets on it.

3. Cover and keep the heat medium-high. Grill for about 3 to 5 minutes on each side. Check the flakiness using a fork. Set aside.

4. In the same grill rack, heat the tortillas for about 40 seconds. Keep the tortillas warm.

5. Divide the fillets according to the number of tortillas, and layer with the cilantro, cabbage and salsa, and then squeeze the lime juice and drizzle some pepper sauce.

6. Fold and serve.

7. You will get 6 servings in the end.

Nutritional Information (per serving)

- Calories- 284

- Fat- 5 g

- Saturated fat- 1 g

- Sodium- 278 mg

- Cholesterol- 24 mg

- Carbohydrate- 26 g

- Protein- 35 g

Lemon and Mint Bulgur Peas

Number of Servings: 4

Ingredients
- Water- 2 cups

- Bulgur- 1 cup

- Chickpeas- 15 ounces or 1 can, rinse and drain

- Fresh peas- 1 cup, thawed

- Fresh mint- ¼ cup, freshly minced

- Fresh parsley- 1/2 cup, freshly minced

- Sun-dried tomatoes- 2 tbsp, no oil

- Olive oil- ¼ cup

- Pepper- ¼ tsp

- Salt- ½ tsp

Steps to Cook

1. In a large saucepan, boil the water and bulgur together. After boiling, decrease the heat and let the bulgur simmer for about 10 to 12 minutes. Make sure you keep the pan covered during this time.

2. Mix in the fresh peas and cook further, keeping the lid covered, for about 4 to 5 minutes.

3. Move the prepared mixture to a large bowl.

4. In the cooked mixture, add all the other ingredients, and stir properly.

5. You can serve this hot or cold.

Nutritional Information (per serving)

- Calories- 380

- Fat- 16 g

- Saturated fat- 2 g

- Sodium- 450 mg

- Cholesterol- 0 mg

- Carbohydrate- 51 g

- Protein- 11 g

Veggie Chicken Wrapped Delight

Number of Servings: 2

Ingredients

- Shelled edamame- 1 cup

For the dressing:

- Olive oil- 2 tbsp

- Orange juice- 2 tbsp

- Ground ginger- ½ tsp

- Sesame oil- 1 tsp

- Pepper- 1/8 tsp

- Salt- ¼ tsp

For the wraps:

- Cucumber- 1 cup, make thin slices

- Baby spinach- 2 cups

- Carrots- ½ cup, shred properly

- Snap peas- 1 cup, freshly chopped

- Chicken breast- 1 cup, cooked and chopped

- Red bell pepper- ½ cup, sweet version, thinly sliced

- Tortillas- 8, 8 inches, whole wheat

Steps to Cook

1. Follow the package directions to cook the edamame. Drain properly, and rinse using cold water.

2. Whisk all the dressing items together and mix.

3. Take out a large bowl to mix all the veggies with the edamame and chicken. Toss this mixture with the prepared dressing.

4. Divide ½ cup mixture portions, and fill it in the tortilla. Fold and roll.

5. Serve 2 wraps as one serving.

Nutritional Information (per serving)

- Calories- 214 (for 1 wrap)

- Fat- 7 g

- Saturated fat- 1 g

- Sodium- 229 mg

- Cholesterol- 13 mg

- Carbohydrate- 28 g

- Protein- 12 g

Tomato, Ricotta and Corn Macaroni

Number of Servings: 6

Ingredients

- Cannellini beans- 1 can of 15 ounces, rinse and drain
- Elbow macaroni- 3 cups, whole wheat, uncooked
- Fresh corn- 1 cup, thawed
- Cherry tomatoes- 2 cups, halved
- Red onion- ½ cup, chopped
- Parmesan cheese- ¼ cup, shredded
- Ricotta cheese- ½ cup, partially skimmed
- Olive oil- 1 tbsp
- Fresh basil- 2 tbsp, freshly minced
- Garlic- 3 cloves, minced
- Dried basil- 2 tsp
- Fresh rosemary- 1 tsp
- Salt- 1 tsp
- Dried rosemary- ½ tsp

- Baby spinach- 3 cups

- Pepper- ½ tsp

- Fresh parsley- chopped

Steps to Cook

1. Follow the instructions given on the macaroni package to cook. Drain, and use cold water to rinse the cooked macaroni properly.

2. In a large bowl, mix together the tomatoes, beans, corn, ricotta, onion, oil, basil, parmesan, ricotta, pepper, rosemary, garlic and salt. Mix everything and add macaroni as well.

3. Combine the whole mixture and add some parsley.

Nutritional Information (per serving)

- Calories- 275

- Fat- 5 g

- Saturated fat- 1 g

- Sodium- 429 mg

- Cholesterol- 7 mg

- Carbohydrate- 46 g

- Protein- 13 g

Pesto Shrimp with Sweetcorn and Avocados

Number of Servings: 4

Ingredients

- Basil leaves- ½ cup, fresh
- Sweet corn- 4, medium-sized, remove husks
- Salt- ½ tsp, divided
- Olive oil- ¼ cup
- Pepper- 1/8 tsp
- Cherry tomatoes- 1½ cups, halved
- Shrimp- 1 pound, peel and devein, uncooked
- Ripe avocado- 1, peel and chop

Steps to Cook

1. Boil the water in a large pot and cook the available corn. This should take about 4 to 5 minutes. Remove and drain. Let the corn cool down during this time.

2. Now, pulse ¼ tsp of salt, oil and basil in a blender.

3. Cut all the corn and set aside. Mix the corn with the pepper, tomatoes and salt. Add the basil mixture and avocado. Stir properly.

4. Use soaked skewers made of wood to thread

the available shrimp. Keep the heat medium-high, and cook for about 2 to 5 minutes.

5. Serve the cooked shrimp with the cooked corn mixture.

6. You will get 4 servings.

Nutritional Information (per serving)

- Calories- 371

- Fat- 22 g

- Saturated fat- 3 g

- Sodium- 450 mg

- Cholesterol- 38 mg

- Carbohydrate- 25 g

- Protein- 23 g

Stuffed Sweet Potato Yogurt Mash

Number of Servings: 2

Ingredients

- Greek yogurt- ½ cup, low-fat, choose coconut yogurt

- Sweet potato- 4, medium-sized

- Apple- 1, chopped

- Maple syrup- 2 tbsp

- Coconut flakes- ¼ cup, unsweetened and toasted

Steps to Cook

1. Prepare your oven by preheating it to 400 degrees. Take out a baking sheet, and line it with foil. Place potatoes on the sheet, and put in the oven. Bake for about 40 to 50 minutes to get tender potatoes.

2. Use a knife to make an "X" shape in every potato. Pulp the boiled potatoes with a small fork.

3. Put all the ingredients together and serve.

Nutritional Information (per serving)

- Calories- 321 (1 stuffed potato)

- Fat- 3 g

- Saturated fat- 2 g

- Sodium- 36 mg

- Cholesterol- 0 mg

- Carbohydrate- 70 g

- Protein- 7 g

Creamy Pistachio Salmon

Number of Servings: 6

Ingredients

- Sour cream- 1/3 cup

- Salmon- 6 fillets

- Pistachios- 2/3 cup, roughly chopped

- Breadcrumbs- 2/3 cup, dried

- Olive oil- 2 tbsp

- Shallot- 1, roughly minced

- Fresh dill- 1 tbsp

- Horseradish- 2 tbsp, ready-to-use

- Pepper flakes- ¼ tsp, crushed

- Orange zest- ½ tsp

- Garlic- 1 clove, finely minced

Steps to Cook

1. Prepare your oven by preheating it to 350 degrees.

2. Place the fillets on a baking pan. No need to grease the pan. Just place the skin side toward the pan's bottom.

3. Coat every fillet with sour cream.

4. Now, you can combine all the other ingredients in one bowl. Mix and place the mixture on top of the fillets.

5. Move to the preheated oven, and bake for about 13 to 15 minutes. Check the readiness of the fish.

6. Serves 6 people.

Nutritional Information (per serving)

- Calories- 376

- Fat- 25 g

- Saturated fat- 5 g

- Sodium- 219 mg

- Cholesterol- 40 mg

- Carbohydrate- 15 g

- Protein- 24 g

Pork Roast Lunch Salad

Number of Servings: 12

Ingredients

1. Apple cider- 1½ cups

2. Loin roast of pork- 1 of 4 pounds, boneless

3. Garlic- 3 cloves, minced

4. Green chilies- 4 ounces, drained and chopped

5. Salt- 1½ tsp

6. Chili powder- 1 tsp

7. Hot sauce- 1½ tsp

8. Ground cumin- ½ tsp

9. Pepper- 1 tsp

10. Chili powder- 1 tsp

11. Salad greens- 12 cups, roughly torn

12. Dried oregano- ½ tsp

13. Tomatoes- 2, chopped

14. Black beans- 1 can of 15 ounces, rinse and drain

15. Corn- 1 cup, frozen or fresh

16. Red onion- 1, chopped

17. Dressing- low-salt

18. Cotija cheese- 1 cup, low-fat

Steps to Cook

1. You will need your slow cooker for this. Place the pork in the cooker.

2. Use a large bowl to mix the green chilies, cider, salt, garlic, chili powder, pepper, sauce, oregano and cumin. Mix properly, and pour it over the pork.

3. Cover the cooker with the lid, and choose a low-pressure setting to cook for about 7 to 8 hours. Make sure the meat gets tender during this time.

4. Now, you can take out the roasted pork from the cooker, and remove all the cooking juices.

5. Use a fork to properly shred the cooked roast.

6. Take out the serving platter, and layer it with the salad greens. Add the shredded pork over the salad greens and top with the tomatoes, black beans, corn, cheese and onion.

7. Drizzle some dressing and serve.

8. You will get 12 servings with this recipe.

Nutritional Information (per serving)

- Calories- 233

- Fat- 8 g

- Saturated fat- 4 g

- Sodium- 321 mg

- Cholesterol- 47 mg

- Carbohydrate- 12 g

- Protein- 28 g

Garlic Chicken with Portobello Mushrooms

Number of Servings: 4

Ingredients

- Pepper- ¼ tsp

- Salt- ½ tsp

- Olive oil- 1 tbsp

- Half chicken breast- 4 pieces, skinless and boneless

- Onion- 1, chopped

- Portobello mushrooms- 2 cups, slices

- Chicken broth- ½ cup, low-sodium

Steps to Cook

1. Use a mallet to flatten the chicken breast pieces. Season with pepper and salt.

2. Use a large skillet and heat the oil, keeping the heat medium-high.

3. Put in the chicken pieces, and cook each side for about 4 to 6 minutes. Set aside, and cover to keep the pieces warm.

4. In the same pan, add the onion and mushroom

pieces. Cook for about 3 to 4 minutes until brown, stirring occasionally. Add the garlic, and cook for 1 minute more. Pour in the low-sodium broth and boil. Stir more, and cook for about 2 minutes to get a slightly thick consistency.

5. Pour over the chicken and serve warm.

6. You will get 4 servings.

Nutritional Information (per serving)

- Calories- 243

- Fat- 7 g

- Saturated fat- 2 g

- Sodium- 381 mg

- Cholesterol- 44 mg

- Carbohydrate- 5 g

- Protein- 36 g

Italian Style Lentils with Artichoke and Kale

Number of Servings: 4

Ingredients

- Dried oregano- ¼ tsp

- Red lentils- 1/2 cup, sort and rinse

- Vegetable broth- 1¼ cups

- Pepper- 1/8 tsp

- Olive oil- 1 tbsp

- Sea salt- ¼ tsp, divided

- Artichoke hearts- 14 ounces of 1 can, packed in water, drain and chop

- Fresh kale- 16 cups, chopped

- Italian seasoning- ½ tsp

- Cooked brown rice- 2 cups

- Romano cheese- 2 tbsp, shredded

Steps to Cook

1. In a medium-sized saucepan, add the oregano, lentils, pepper, broth and about ½ tsp of salt. Boil this mixture.

2. Keeping the pan covered, simmer the lentils for about 13 to 15 minutes. This time will allow the liquid to become absorbed, and then you can switch off the heat and set this aside.

3. Use a large stockpot to heat the oil, keeping the heat medium, then include the kale, along with the rest of the salt. Cover and cook for about 3 to 5 minutes. Stir from time to time. Add the

artichoke hearts, Italian seasoning and garlic. Give 3 more minutes to cook, stirring.

4. Switch off the heat, and mix in the shredded cheese.

5. Serve the lentils and kale with 1 cup of brown, cooked rice.

6. You will get 4 servings.

Nutritional Information (per serving)

- Calories- 321

- Fat- 6 g

- Saturated fat- 2 g

- Sodium- 661 mg

- Cholesterol- 1 mg

- Carbohydrate- 53 g

- Protein- 15 g

Pepper Quinoa with Turkey Sausage

Number of Servings: 2

Ingredients

- Quinoa- ¾ cup, rinsed

- Vegetable stock- 1 1/2 cups

116

- Red bell pepper- 1, chopped

- Turkey sausage- 1 pound, remove the casings

- Sweet onion- ¾ cup, roughly chopped

- Green bell pepper- 1, chopped

- Garam masala- ¼ tsp

- Garlic- 1 clove, finely minced

- Pepper- ¼ tsp

- Salt- 1/8 tsp

Steps to Cook

1. Put the vegetable stock in a saucepan along with the quinoa and boil, then simmer for about 13 to 15 minutes, keeping the pan covered. Set aside.

2. Cook the sausage in a large skillet and crumble simultaneously. Include the onion and all peppers, and cook for about 9 to 10 minutes. Add in the seasonings and garlic to cook for a further extra minute. Keep stirring during this time.

3. After getting the fragrance of garlic, include quinoa and cook for 2 minutes, stirring.

4. Serve.

Nutritional Information (per serving)

- Calories- 261

- Fat- 9 g

- Saturated fat- 2 g

- Sodium- 760 mg

- Cholesterol- 42 mg

- Carbohydrate- 28 g

- Protein- 17 g

The DASH Diet Meal Recipes for Dinner

Creamy Risotto with a Plum Tomato Roast

Number of Servings: 8

Ingredients

- Olive oil- 2 tbsp, extra-virgin

- Plum tomatoes- 10, make wedges

- Black pepper- ½ tsp, freshly ground, divided

- Salt- ½ tsp, divided

- Water- 3 cups

- Vegetable stock- 4 cups, reduced-sodium

- Pearl barley- 2 cups

- Shallots- 2, chopped

- Italian parsley- 3 tbsp, chopped

- Fresh basil- 3 tbsp, chopped

- Parmesan cheese- ½ cup, shredded

- Thyme- 1½ tbsp, freshly chopped

Steps to Cook

1. Heat your oven to 450 degrees F.

2. Take a baking sheet, and layer the tomatoes on it. Pour on the oil, and sprinkle ¼ tsp of salt along with some pepper. Mix carefully. Roast the tomatoes to make them soft and light brown. This should take about 20 to 30 minutes.

3. In a large saucepan, boil the water and vegetable stock together. Then, decrease the heat, and let it simmer.

4. Take another saucepan and heat the olive oil, keeping the heat medium. Add the shallots and cook for about 1 to 3 minutes. Include the barley and cook for about 1 to 2 minutes, stirring.

5. Now, mix about ½ cup of the stock in the barley mixture and cook, stirring, until the liquid is absorbed. Then, add more stock and repeat this process until you finish the whole stock mixture. This should take about 4 to 5 minutes after which you will have a tender barley mixture.

6. Switch off the heat and mix the parsley, basil, tomatoes, cheese and thyme. Adjust the pepper and salt and combine properly.

7. Serve with the roasted tomato pieces.

8. You will get 8 servings.

Nutritional Information (per serving)

- Calories- 287

- Fat- 7 g

- Saturated fat- 2 g

- Sodium- 288 mg

- Cholesterol- 5 mg

- Carbohydrate- 45 g

- Protein- 11 g

Lean Beef and Vegetable Stew

Number of Servings: 4

Ingredients

- Canola oil- 2 tsp

- Beef- 1 pound, lean meat, round steak

- Celery- 1 cup, roughly diced

- Yellow onions- 2 cups

- Sweet potato- ½ cup, roughly diced

- Roma tomatoes- 1 cup, roughly diced

- Mushrooms- ½ cup, roughly diced

- White potato- ½ cup, roughly diced with skin

- Garlic- 4 cloves, chopped

- Carrot- 1 cup, roughly diced

- Uncooked barley- ¼ cup

- Kale- 1 cup, roughly chopped

- Balsamic vinegar- 1 tsp

- Wine vinegar- ¼ cup

- Dried sage- 1 tsp, crushed

- Vegetable stock- 3 cups, reduced-sodium

- Fresh thyme- 1 tsp, minced

- Dried oregano- 1 tbsp

- Fresh parsley- 1 tbsp

- Black pepper- according to taste

- Dried rosemary- 1 tsp, minced

Steps to Cook

1. Choose a medium heat when preheating your grill. Then, grill the beef steak for about 6 to 7 minutes on each side. Only brown, don't let it get overcooked. Set aside.

2. Choose a large-sized stockpot to cook all the vegetables for about 9 to 10 minutes, until tender, keeping the heat medium-high.

3. After cooking the vegetables, add the barley in the same mixture, and cook for an extra 4 to 5 minutes.

4. Use a paper towel to dry the meat, and then cut the steak into small pieces and add into the stockpot. Top it with herbs, stock, vinegar and spices.

5. Simmer for about 60 minutes to get a stew-like consistency.

6. You will get 4 servings.

Nutritional Information (per serving)

- Calories- 389

- Fat- 9 g

- Saturated fat- 2 g

- Sodium- 166 mg

- Cholesterol- 34 mg

- Carbohydrate- 35 g

- Protein- 42 g

Creamy Rigatoni Noodles with Cooked Broccoli

Number of Servings: 2

Ingredients

- Broccoli florets- 2 cups

- Rigatoni noodles- 1/3 pound

- Olive oil- 2 tsp

- Parmesan cheese- 2 tbsp

- Black pepper- according to taste, freshly ground

- Minced garlic- 2 tsp

Steps to Cook

1. Fill a large pot with water. Add the pasta and submerge completely. Cook for about 11 to 15 minutes to get tender noodles. Drain the noodles completely.

2. Steam the broccoli for about 8 to 10 minutes, keeping the pot covered.

3. Now, mix the cooked noodles with the steamed broccoli, and add the olive oil, garlic and cheese. Add pepper to tast and serve.

4. You will get two servings with this recipe.

Nutritional Information (per serving)

- Calories- 355

- Fat- 7 g

- Saturated fat- 2 g

- Sodium- 111 mg

- Cholesterol- 4 mg

- Carbohydrate- 63 g

- Protein- 14 g

Caper Cooked Cod

Number of Servings: 6

Ingredients

- Lemons- 2

- Cod- 4 fillets, every fillet should have 6 ounces of weight

- Hot water- 1 cup

- Bouillon granules- 1 tsp, reduced-sodium, choose the chicken flavor

- All-purpose flour- 1 tbsp, plain

- Soft butter- 1 tbsp

- Capers- 4 tsp, rinse and drain

Steps to Cook

1. Preheat the oven to 350 degrees F.

2. Take four square pieces of foil and spray them with cooking grease.

3. Place the cod fillets onto the foil pieces. Cut and squeeze the lemon over the fillets.

4. Cover the fillets with the foil, and seal properly.

5. Move the sealed fillets to the preheated oven and bake for about 18 to 20 minutes. Use a fork to check the readiness of the fish.

6. During this time, you can prepare the boillon granules in a small-sized bowl by dissolving in hot water. Set aside.

7. In a different bowl, you can mix the flour and butter. Cook this mixture in a pan to melt the butter, stirring. Add the bouillon and cook for longer to get a thick consistency. Finally, include the capers and switch off the heat.

8. When your fish is ready, serve by pouring the prepared mixture over the fillets.

Nutritional Information (per serving)

- Calories- 168

- Fat- 4 g

- Saturated fat- 2 g

- Sodium- 203 mg

- Cholesterol- 31 mg

- Carbohydrate- 2 g

- Protein- 31 g

Avocado, Tomato and Corn Tamales

Number of Servings: 6

Ingredients

- Corn kernels- 3 cups, frozen or fresh, thawed

- Corn husks- 18, and more, dried

- Lukewarm water- ½ cup

- Masa harina- 2 cups

- Salt- ¼ tsp

- Baking powder- 1 tsp

- Canola oil- 3 tbsp

- Bell pepper- green- ¼ cup, red- ¼ cup, all diced

- Pepper flakes- 1/8 tsp

- Yellow onion- 2 tbsp, diced

For the sauce:

- Tomatoes- 4, chopped

- Avocado- ¼ cup, roughly chopped

- Fresh cilantro- 2 tbsp, chopped

- Lime juice- 1 tbsp

- Salt- ¼ tsp

- Jalapeno pepper- ½ tsp, seeded and minced

Steps to Cook

1. Soak the corn husks in water for about 8 to 10 minutes. This will soften them. Drain and properly rinse. Use a paper towel to pat dry the husks before setting aside.

2. Place about 2½ cups of corn kernels into your food processor. Make a puree.

3. In a large bowl, add the masa harina, corn, corn paste, water, oil, ¼ of salt, and baking powder. Blend properly with a wooden spoon. Set aside.

4. In a non-stick pan, fry the bell peppers, the remaining corn kernels, and onion. Cook for about 7 to 8 minutes, keeping the heat on medium. Mix the pepper flakes, and switch off the heat.

5. Now, you can start filling the prepared mixture in the corn husks. Each husk should get about 3 tbsp of the mixture. Use your hand to adjust the thickness, and add the vegetable mixture as well. Each filling can have about 1 tbsp of the veggie mix. Overlap the husks, and use a husk strip to seal each packet. Do the same with all the wraps.

6. Fill the bottom of the pot with water, and place in a basket for steaming. Layer the basket with the prepared tamales wraps. Cover and steam for about 55 to 60 minutes. Check and increase the water level, if required.

7. In a small-sized bowl, you can mix the avocados, lime juice, tomatoes, cilantro, salt and jalapenos.

8. Serve the tamales with the prepared sauce.

9. You will get 6 servings in the end.

Nutritional Information (per serving)

- Calories- 335

- Fat- 11 g

- Saturated fat- 1 g

- Sodium- 338 mg

- Cholesterol- 0 mg

- Carbohydrate- 52 g

- Protein- 7 g

Mustard Black-Eyed Peas

Number of Servings: 8

Ingredients
- Black-eyed peas- 2 cups, choose dried ones

- Water- 3 cups

- Unsalted tomatoes- 2 cups, crushed

- Chicken bouillon- 1 tsp, reduced-sodium

- Celery- 2 stalks, properly chopped

- Onion- 1, properly chopped

- Garlic- 3 tsp, minced

- Ground ginger- ¼ tsp

- Dry mustard- ½ tsp

- Bay leaf- 1

- Cayenne pepper- ¼ tsp

- Parsley- ½ cup, roughly chopped

Steps to Cook
1. Keeping the heat high, boil the black-eyed peas in a water-filled saucepan. This will take about

10 to 20 minutes. Then, cover the pan, and set aside to rest for about 45 to 50 minutes.

2. Drain the water from the pan. Then, include run fresh water over the peas and add the tomatoes, bouillon, onion, mustard, garlic, ginger, celery, bay leaf and cayenne pepper. Stir until boiling, then decrease the heat to simmer for about 2 hours. Make sure you cover the pan and stir the mixture occasionally. If required, include more water to cover the peas.

3. Discard the bay leaf and transfer the mixture into a large serving bowl. Serve warm.

4. You will get about 8 servings.

Nutritional Information (per serving)
- Calories- 173

- Fat- 1 g

- Saturated fat- 0.5 g

- Sodium- 43 mg

- Cholesterol- 0 mg

- Carbohydrate- 32 g

- Protein- 11 g

Garlic Fettuccine with Basil and Clams

Number of Servings: 6

Ingredients

- Minced garlic- 2 tbsp

- Uncooked fettuccine- 10 ounces

- Corn kernels- 2 cups, frozen or fresh

- Tomatoes- 2, seeds removed and chopped

- Olive oil- 1 tbsp

- White wine- ½ cup

- Clams- 2 cans of 4 ounces, drained

- Fresh basil- 4 tbsp, freshly chopped

- Black pepper- according to taste, ground

- Salt- ¼ tsp

Steps to Cook

1. Take a large pot, fill with water and boil. Then, submerge the fettuccine pasta in it to boil for about 5 to 8 minutes, or follow the package directions. Drain to remove the water.

2. Use a large-sized saucepan to boil a mixture of corn, tomatoes, garlic, olive oil, basil and wine. Keep the pan covered during this time. Just

stir occasionally.

3. Now, decrease the heat, and add the pasta and clams. Coat and flavor with pepper and salt.

4. Serve warm.

5. You will get 6 servings with this recipe.

Nutritional Information (per serving)

- Calories- 316

- Fat- 4 g

- Saturated fat- 0.5 g

- Sodium- 147 mg

- Cholesterol- 19 mg

- Carbohydrate- 52 g

- Protein- 18 g

Brown Rice with a Tomato Herb Sauce

Number of Servings: 6

Ingredients

- Kalamata olives- 4, sliced

- Plum tomatoes- 4 cups, roughly chopped

- Capers- 1½ tsp, rinse and properly drain

- Green olives- 4, sliced

- Olive oil- 1 tbsp

- Minced garlic- 1 tbsp

- Minced parsley- 1 tbsp, fresh

- Chopped basil- ¼ cup, fresh

- Pepper flakes- 1/8 tsp

- Brown rice- 3 cups, steam cooked

Steps to Cook

1. In a large-sized bowl, mix the olives, tomatoes, garlic, capers and oil. Add the basil as well as the pepper flakes. Stir properly to get the desired consistency.

2. Cover the bowl, and let rest for about 30 to 40 minutes. Stir from time to time.

3. Cook your brown rice during this time.

4. Serve the brown rice with the prepared mixture on top.

5. You will get 6 servings.

Nutritional Information (per serving)

- Calories- 250

- Fat- 6 g

- Saturated fat- 1 g

- Sodium- 182 mg

- Cholesterol- 0 mg

- Carbohydrate- 44 g

- Protein- 5 g

Mixed-Fruit Stuffed Turkey Breasts

Number of Servings: 12

Ingredients
- Turkey breast- 5-pound piece, whole and bone-in

For the rub:

- Fresh thyme- 2 tbsp, chopped

- Fresh rosemary- 2 tbsp, chopped

- Olive oil- 2 tbsp

For the stuffing:

- Apple- 1, skin removed and sliced

- Onion- 1, thin slices

- Dried cranberries- ¼ cup

- Pear- 1, skin removed and sliced

For the glazing:

- Brown sugar- 1 tbsp

- Apple juice- 2 cups, divided

- Olive oil- 1 tbsp

- Brown mustard- 1 tbsp

Steps to Cook

1. Prepare your oven by preheating it to 325 degrees F.

2. Place the whole turkey in a large roasting pan. Make sure you keep the skin portion face up.

3. In another bowl, mix all the herbs along with the oil to create a paste.

4. Use your fingers to create a large space between the turkey meat and its skin. Now, put ½ of the prepared paste in that space; plus, drizzle the rest all over the outer part of the turkey.

5. In another bowl, combine the onion slices and fruits, then stuff the created space in the breast with this fruit mixture as well.

6. In your roasting pan, add half of the available apple juice and place the turkey breast. Roast about 2 hours, keeping the heat medium-high. Check to ensure that the internal meat temperature reaches 165 degrees F.

7. During this time, you can prepare the glaze by

mixing the brown sugar, the apple juice, olive oil and mustard. Heat this mixture at a high temperature, and simmer to get a thick consistency.

8. During the last 40 minutes of the turkey cooking, you can add some of the glaze to baste.

9. Let the turkey rest for about 10 to 15 minutes, and then pour the rest of the glazing mixture over it and carve.

10. Serve warm.

11. You will get about 12 servings.

Nutritional Information (per serving)

- Calories- 350

- Fat- 14 g

- Saturated fat- 4 g

- Sodium- 117 mg

- Cholesterol- 41 mg

- Carbohydrate- 15 g

- Protein- 41 g

Asian-Style Ginger Salmon

Number of Servings: 2

Ingredients

- Soy sauce- 1 tbsp, low-sodium

- Sesame oil- 1 tbsp

- Vinegar- 1 tbsp, choose rice wine

- Ginger- 1 tbsp, freshly minced

- Salmon- 4 fillets, every fillet should weigh 4 ounces

Steps to Cook

1. Use a glass dish to mix the soy sauce, sesame oil, vinegar and ginger. Place the salmon in the dish, and coat with the mixture in all directions. Leave in your refrigerator for about 50 to 60 minutes. After 30 minutes of refrigeration, turn the salmon fillets over once.

2. When cooking, keep the heat medium-high, and grease a pan lightly with the oil. Grill each side for about 4 to 5 minutes. Use a knife to make a cut, and see if the flesh looks opaque or not.

3. Serve with the cilantro, and garnish with the lemon wedges.

Nutritional Information (per serving)

- Calories- 185

- Fat- 9 g

- Saturated fat- 2 g

- Sodium- 113 mg

- Cholesterol- 47 mg

- Carbohydrate- 1 g

- Protein- 26 g

Orange Chicken with Olives and Celery

Number of Servings: 4

Ingredients

- Garlic- 4 cloves, finely minced

- Wine vinegar- ½ cup, choose red wine

- Red onion- 1 tbsp, properly chopped

- Olive oil- 1 tbsp, extra-virgin

- Black pepper- according to taste, cracked

- Celery- 1 tbsp, properly chopped

- Garlic- 2 cloves, for the salad

- Chicken breasts- 4 pieces, each should weigh 4 ounces, boneless and skinless

- Black olives- 16, ripe

- Lettuce- 8 cups, wash and dry

- Orange- 2 navels, peel and slice

Steps to Cook

1. Use a small-sized bowl to mix together the garlic, vinegar, onion, olive oil, pepper and celery. Get an even consistency by stirring thoroughly. This will work as your dressing. You can refrigerate in a covered bowl for the time being.

2. Prepare your grill for high-heat cooking. Grease the grilling rack with some cooking spray. Place the greased rack about 5 to 6 inches into the grill. Coat the chicken pieces with the available cloves of garlic. Brown each side in the grill for about 4 to 5 minutes on every side.

3. Shift to a wooden board and cut into pieces after letting it rest for 8 minutes.

4. Arrange servings with the orange slices, olives, lettuce and chicken pieces. Use your prepared dressing to drizzle all over the chicken and lettuce.

5. You will get 4 healthy servings with this

recipe.

Nutritional Information (per serving)

- Calories- 237

- Fat- 9 g

- Saturated fat- 1 g

- Sodium- 199 mg

- Cholesterol- 43 mg

- Carbohydrate- 12 g

- Protein- 27 g

Snapper Coconut Curry

Number of Servings: 4

Ingredients

- Black pepper- 1 tsp

- Coconut extract- ½ tsp

- Turmeric- 1 tbsp

- Fennel seed- ½ tsp

- Cumin- 1 tsp

- Coriander- 1 tsp

- Skim milk- 1 cup

- Paprika- 1 tsp

- Canola oil- 1 tsp

- Cornstarch- 1 tsp

- Poblano pepper- 1, sliced

- Fresh ginger- 2 tbsp, minced

- Bok choy- 2 cups, slices

- Bell pepper- 1 cup, red one, sliced

- Celery- 2 cups, slices

- Garlic- 2 cloves, minced

- Snapper- 4 fillets, each fillet should weigh about 6 ounces

Steps to Cook

1. In a large bowl, mix all the spices, along with the milk, cornstarch and coconut extract. Set aside.

2. Use a large-sized skillet to heat some oil, keeping the heat medium-high. Add the vegetables, and sauté for about 3 to 4 minutes until the vegetables are a little tender and lightly golden brown.

3. With the sautéed vegetables, add the mixture of milk, coconut and spices. Stir properly, and

heat thoroughly without boiling. Set aside.

4. Grease a grilling pan, and grill all the fish fillets to reach about 145 degrees F of internal temperature.

5. Serve 1 plate with one fillet and vegetable curry.

6. You will get four servings.

Nutritional Information (per serving)

- Calories- 295

- Fat- 7 g

- Saturated fat- 1 g

- Sodium- 246 mg

- Cholesterol- 43 mg

- Carbohydrate- 18 g

- Protein- 40 g

Honey Paprika Chicken

Number of Servings: 2

Ingredients

- Paprika- 1 tsp

- Saltine crackers- 8, every piece should

measure 2 inches

- Honey- 4 tsp

- Chicken breasts- 2 pieces, each piece should weigh 4 ounces

Steps to Cook

1. Prepare your oven by preheating it to a temperature of 375 degrees F.

2. Use a cooking spray to grease your baking dish.

3. In a small-sized bowl, crush all the saltine crackers, and mix with paprika.

4. In a different bowl, mix the chicken pieces with the honey. Coat properly and add the mixture of crackers and paprika. Mix properly.

5. Place the coated chicken pieces into the greased baking pan. Cook about 22 to 30 minutes until the chicken is browned.

6. Serve warm.

7. You will get two servings in the end.

Nutritional Information (per serving)

- Calories- 219

- Fat- 3 g

- Saturated fat- 1 g

- Sodium- 187 mg

- Cholesterol- 46 mg

- Carbohydrate- 21 g

- Protein- 27 g

Vegetable-Packed Chicken

Number of Servings: 6

Ingredients
- Zucchini- ½ cup, chopped

- Chicken breast- 1, boneless and skinless, the piece should weigh 3 ounces

- Onion- ¼ cup, chopped

- Potato- ½ cup, chopped after scrubbing

- Garlic powder- 1/8 tsp

- Mushrooms- ¼ cup, slices

- Baby carrots- ¼ cup, slices

- Oregano- ¼ tsp

Steps to Cook
1. Preheat your oven to a temperature of 350 degrees F.

2. Cut aluminum foil into 12 inch pieces. Fold and unfold this foil in half, and then grease the surface with the cooking spray.

3. Place the chicken pieces right in the middle of the greased surface. Layer with potato, zucchini, carrots, mushrooms and onions. Spread some oregano and garlic powder over the vegetables and the chicken.

4. Wrap to make a small packet, and seal tightly.

5. Place this sealed packet on your baking sheet and bake for about 40 to 50 minutes. Check chicken with a fork, and then take out.

Nutritional Information (per serving)

- Calories- 207

- Fat- 2.5 g

- Saturated fat- 0.5 g

- Sodium- 72 mg

- Cholesterol- 42 mg

- Carbohydrate- 23 g

- Protein- 23 g

Mango and Pineapple Low-Fat Pizza

Number of Servings: 4

Ingredients

- Onion- ½ cup, finely minced

- Bell peppers- 1 cup, a mixture of green and red, chopped

- Pineapple tidbits- ½ cup

- Mango- ½ cup, peel and remove seed, chopped

- Cilantro- ½ cup, freshly chopped

- Lime juice- 1 tbsp

- Whole grain crust for pizza- 1, about 12 inches, ready-to-use

Steps to Cook

1. Prepare your oven by preheating to a temperature of 425 degrees F.

2. Use cooking spray to grease a round baking pan.

3. Use a small-sized bowl to mix the onions, peppers, mango, lime juice, cilantro and pineapple. Set aside.

4. Roll and set the dough in your greased pan.

Shift to the preheated oven and cook for 12 to 16 minutes.

5. Take out the crust, and layer it with the pineapple and mango mixture prepared earlier. Bake for about 6 to 9 minutes until fruit is browned.

6. Cut about 8 slices and enjoy.

7. You will get 4 servings.

Nutritional Information (per serving)

- Calories- 250

- Fat- 4 g

- Saturated fat- 1.5 g

- Sodium- 354 mg

- Cholesterol- 0 mg

- Carbohydrate- 45 g

- Protein- 8 g

Butternut Squash Pasta

Number of Servings: 6

Ingredients

- Olive oil- 2 tbsp, separated

- Butternut squash- 1, split and remove seed. It should weigh 2 pounds

- Linguine pasta- 12 ounces, choose whole wheat

- Black pepper- according to taste

- Sage leaves- 8, strip cut

- Vegetable broth- 1½ cups, low-sodium

- Bell pepper- ½ cup, red one, chopped

- Yellow onion- ¼ cup, chopped

- Cider vinegar- 1 tbsp

- Garlic- 2 cloves, minced

- Ground nutmeg- 1/8 tsp

Steps to Cook

1. Preheat your oven to a temperature of 400 degrees F.

2. Use half of the oil to coat the squash. Also, season with some pepper. Give this about 50 to 70 minutes of roasting in the oven, then let it cool down.

3. Pour water into a large pot and boil. Cook the pasta according to the instructions on the packaging.

4. In your blender, puree the cooked squash to get a smooth consistency. Also, add the broth

149

and keep blending. If desired, you can also include some water. Make sure the consistency is not too light.

5. In a small-sized skillet, heat the rest of the oil keeping the heat medium-high. Then, add the sage to cook for about ½ a minute. Add the red pepper, onion, as well as the garlic. Cook this mixture for about 4 to 6 minutes.

6. Add the squash puree in the vegetable mixture, along with the nutmeg, pepper, and vinegar.

7. Finally, add the cooked pasta and coat with the mixture thoroughly.

8. Serves 6 people.

Nutritional Information (per serving)

- Calories- 255

- Fat- 7 g

- Saturated fat- 2 g

- Sodium- 206 mg

- Cholesterol- 33 mg

- Carbohydrate- 38 g

- Protein- 10 g

Raisin and Spinach Pasta

Number of Servings: 3

Ingredients

- Olive oil- 2 tbsp

- Pasta- 8 ounces, bow tie, dry

- Garbanzos- 10 ounces, canned, rinse and drain

- Garlic- 4 cloves, crush

- Golden raisins- ½ cup

- Chicken broth- ½ cup, no salt

- Parmesan cheese- 2 tbsp, shredded

- Spinach- 4 cups, freshly chopped

- Black peppercorns- according to taste, cracked

Steps to Cook

1. Boil water in a large-sized pot. Keep the water level about ¾ high in the pot.

2. Put the pasta into the boiling water, and cook according to the instructions on the package. This should take about 11 to 15 minutes, then drain, and set aside the pasta.

3. Use a large-sized skillet to mix the garlic and oil, keeping the heat medium. Add the

garbanzos along with the vegetable broth. Cook for about 1 minute, stirring, then add the spinach and raisins. Heat a little bit to wilt the spinach. This should only take about 2 to 3 minutes.

4. Divide the cooked pasta into three servings, and pour on the prepared sauce along with the peppercorns and cheese.

5. Serve.

Nutritional Information (per serving)

- Calories- 283

- Fat- 7 g

- Saturated fat- 1 g

- Sodium- 130 mg

- Cholesterol- 1 mg

- Carbohydrate- 44 g

- Protein- 11 g

Grilled Vegetable Pasta

Number of Servings: 4

Ingredients

- Fresh tomatoes- 10 large, peel and dice

- Olive oil- 2 tbsp, separated, extra-virgin

- Minced garlic- ½ tsp

- Fresh basil- 1 tbsp

- Chopped onion- 2 tbsp

- Dried oregano- ½ tsp

- Sugar- 1 tsp

- Red peppers- 2, slices

- Black pepper- 1/8 tsp, freshly ground

- Zucchini- 1, slices

- Yellow squash- 1 whole, sliced

- Spaghetti- 8 ounces, choose whole wheat

Steps to Cook

1. Use a large skillet to prepare your sauce. Start by heating 1 tbsp of oil, keeping the heat medium-high. Add the garlic, tomatoes, basil, onions, pepper, oregano and sugar. Cook, then simmer for about 20 to 30 minutes to get a thick sauce, stirring.

2. Prepare your grill by coating the grilling rack with cooking spray.

3. Coat the squash, red peppers, sweet onion and zucchini with the rest of the olive oil, then carefully place all these veggies on the greased

153

rack, and grill for about 7 to 8 minutes. This will give you tender grilled vegetables.

4. Cook your pasta in boiling water for about 9 to 12 minutes, or you can follow the package directions. Remove the water and drain properly.

5. Serve the pasta with the vegetables, and the prepared sauce.

6. You will get 4 servings.

Nutritional Information (per serving)

- Calories- 361

- Fat- 5 g

- Saturated fat- 5 g

- Sodium- 315 mg

- Cholesterol- 0 mg

- Carbohydrate- 66 g

- Protein- 13 g

Garlic Cornmeal with Broccoli Mushrooms and Zucchini

Number of Servings: 4

Ingredients

- Water- 4 cups

- Cornmeal- 1 cup, ground

- Mushrooms- 1 cup, freshly sliced

- Garlic- 1 tsp, chopped

- Broccoli florets- 1 cup

- Onion slices- 1 cup

- Parmesan cheese- 2 tbsp, grated

- Zucchini slices- 1 cup

- Oregano- according to taste, freshly chopped

Steps to Cook

1. Preheat your oven to get a temperature of 350 degrees F.

2. Coat a microwave-safe dish with cooking spray.

3. Mix the cornmeal with the garlic and water in the greased dish. Bake this mixture without covering for about 35 to 45 minutes. The

mixture will start leaving the sides of the container.

4. During this time, you can use a non-stick pan to fry the onions and mushrooms. Grease a little and include the vegetables, keeping the heat medium. This should take about 4 to 6 minutes.

5. Fill some water in a pot. Choose a basket for steaming. Layer the zucchini and broccoli in the basket for steaming over the pot.

6. Cover and let the veggies steam for about 3 to 4 minutes.

7. Now, serve the cornmeal with the vegetables, and top with parmesan and herbs.

8. You will get 4 servings.

Nutritional Information (per serving)

- Calories- 178

- Fat- 1 g

- Saturated fat- 0.2 g

- Sodium- 55 mg

- Cholesterol- 2 mg

- Carbohydrate- 34 g

- Protein- 6 g

Herbes de Provence Pork

Number of Servings: 2

Ingredients

- Black pepper- according to taste, ground

- Pork tenderloin- 8 ounces, lean meat, make 6 pieces after trimming the fat

- White wine- ¼ cup, dried white wine

- Herbes de Provence- ½ tsp

Steps to Cook

1. Use black pepper to season the pork pieces. Use a mallet to adjust the thickness of the pieces. You need to make about ¼ inch thick pieces.

2. Use a large non-stick pan to fry these meat pieces, keeping the heat medium-high. This should take about 1 to 3 minutes on each side.

3. Remove the meat from the heat, and spread the Herbes de Provence.

4. Now, boil the wine in the pan, and pour it all over the meat.

5. Serve warm.

6. You will get 2 servings.

Nutritional Information (per serving)

- Calories- 120

- Fat- 2 g

- Saturated fat- 1 g

- Sodium- 62 mg

- Cholesterol- 44 mg

- Carbohydrate- 1 g

- Protein- 24 g

Anchovy Prawns with Herbs

Number of Servings: 4

Ingredients

- Prawns- 1 ¼ pounds, peel and devein

- Olive oil- 2 tbsp

- White wine- 2 tbsp, dry

- Black pepper- ½ tsp, freshly ground

- Sun-dried tomatoes- ¼ cup, drain and chop

- Tomatoes- 4, peel and remove seeds, dice

- Nicoise olives- ¼ cup, pitted and chopped

- Garlic- 3 cloves, minced

- Anchovy- 2 fillets, rinse and chop

- Capers- 1 tbsp, rinse and chop

- Parsley- 1 tbsp, freshly chopped

- Lemon zest- 1 tbsp, grated

- Basil- 1 tbsp, freshly chopped

Steps to Cook

1. Use a large enough frying pan and heat the oil, keeping the heat medium-high. Put in the prawns, along with the pepper, and cook for 2 to 3 minutes. Turn all the prawns and cook for another 1 or 2 minutes. This will make them pink on both sides. Then, you can move them to a large bowl.

2. Use the wine to deglaze the pan, then add the garlic and sun-dried pieces of tomatoes as well as the fresh tomato pieces. Reduce the heat, and let the mixture simmer for about 2 to 4 minutes.

3. Add all the other ingredients left, and blend the flavors with 2 minutes of cooking.

4. Mix in the cooked prawns and coat properly.

5. Serve warm.

6. You will get 4 servings with this recipe.

Nutritional Information (per serving)

- Calories- 218

- Fat- 5 g

- Saturated fat- 1 g

- Sodium- 379 mg

- Cholesterol- 49 mg

- Carbohydrate- 10 g

- Protein- 31 g

Healthy Vegetable and Lentils Bowl

Number of Servings: 6

Ingredients

- Red onion- 1 cup, roughly chopped

- Canola oil- 2 tsp

- Chili pepper- 1, minced

- Bell pepper- 2 cups, roughly chopped

- Sweet potato- 1 cup, chopped

- Garlic- 2 cloves, minced

- Brown rice- 1 cup

- Tomato- 1 cup, diced

- Red lentils- ½ cup

- Green lentils- ½ cup

- Ground pepper- 1 tbsp, freshly ground

- Ground cumin- 1 tbsp

- Vegetable stock- 2 cups, low-sodium

- Wine vinegar- 1 tbsp

- Chopped kale- 4 cups

- Water- 2 cups

- Fresh cilantro- 2 tbsp, minced

- Black beans- 1 cup, cooked

Steps to Cook

1. Heat the canola oil in a pan, keeping the heat medium-high.

2. Add the peppers, onion, sweet potato, tomato and garlic. Cook this mixture for about 12 to 16 minutes to get translucent onion pieces.

3. Now, include the spices, lentils, water and the stock. Boil, and then decrease the heat to simmer for about 40 to 50 minutes. Keep the pan covered during this time.

4. When ready to serve, include the cilantro, cooked beans and kale with the mixture. Use the lemon wedges to garnish.

5. You will get 6 servings.

Nutritional Information (per serving)

- Calories- 376

- Fat- 5 g

- Saturated fat- 0.9 g

- Sodium- 67 mg

- Cholesterol- 0 mg

- Carbohydrate- 68 g

- Protein- 18 g

Beef Kebabs with Yogurt Sauce

Number of Servings: 4

Ingredients

- Lemon juice- 2 tbsp, fresh

- Yellow onions- 2, roughly chopped

- Lean beef- 1 ½ pounds, ground

- Bulgur- 2 cups, choose fine-grind

162

- Garlic- 2 cloves, minced

- Pine nuts- ¼ cup, finely chopped

- Ground cumin- 1 tsp

- Salt- ½ tsp

- Cardamom- ½ tsp, ground

- Black pepper- ½ tsp, freshly ground

- Cinnamon- ½ tsp, ground

- Wooden skewers- 16, water-soaked

For the sauce:

- Tahini- ¼ cup

- Plain yogurt- 2 cups, no fat

- Dry mustard- 2 tsp

- Lemon zest- 2 tbsp, grated

- Cilantro- 2 tbsp, freshly chopped

Steps to Cook

1. Make a puree of onions in your blender. Press this puree, using a spatula, to separate the juice and solids. Remove the solids, and collect all the onion juice.

2. Into the juice of the onion, add the lemon juice, as well as water to prepare a liquid.

3. Use a large bowl to mix the bulgur with the prepared onion and lemon juice combination. Cook this mixture about 9 to 12 minutes, and then include the pine nuts, beef, salt, garlic, cinnamon, cumin, pepper and cardamom. Mix properly.

4. Measure about 1/3 cup of the mixture for every kebab. You can make about 16 links of beef sausage and thread them one-by-one to skewers. Add water to avoid crumbliness in the mixture. Refrigerate all the prepared sausages in a covered bowl.

5. Prepare your grill and the rack for cooking. Use a cooking spray for greasing the rack.

6. Mix the tahini, yogurt, mustard and lemon zest in a small-sized bowl. Cover and let it cool down in your refrigerator.

7. Now, grill the kebabs by placing them on the rack of the grill. Turn occasionally, and brown for about 7 to 8 minutes.

8. Serve with the yogurt sauce and cilantro.

9. You will get 8 servings.

Nutritional Information (per serving)

- Calories- 372

- Fat- 12 g

- Saturated fat- 1.5 g

- Sodium- 5 mg

- Cholesterol- 5 mg

- Carbohydrate- 4 g

- Protein- 31 g

Broccoli and Mushroom Calzone

Number of Servings: 4

Ingredients

- Spinach- ½ cup, finely chopped

- Asparagus stalks- 3, pieces

- Mushrooms- ½ cup, finely sliced

- Broccoli- ½ cup, finely chopped

- Olive oil- 2 tsp, divided

- Minced garlic- 2 tbsp

- Tomato- 1, sliced

- Bread dough- ½ pound, whole-wheat, frozen then thawed

- Pizza sauce- 2/3 cup

- Mozzarella- ½ cup, part-skim, shredded

Steps to Cook

1. Prepare your oven by heating to a temperature of 400 degrees F.

2. Use a cooking spray to coat the sheet used for baking.

3. Use a large bowl to mix together the spinach, asparagus, mushrooms, garlic and broccoli.

4. Add 1 tsp of olive oil to toss properly.

5. Using a non-stick pan, cook the vegetable mixture, keeping the heat medium-high. This should not take more than 3 to 7 minutes. Keep stirring and then leave aside to rest.

6. Flour a wooden surface to make quarter pieces of the dough. Make circles of every piece.

7. Use your rolling pin to make thin oval shapes with every dough piece.

8. Spread the vegetables, tomato and cheese equally in the ½ portion of the oval piece. Use water to wet the sides of the oval pieces and seal them properly.

9. Carefully move the calzones to the greased baking sheet, and brush all of them with the rest of the olive oil.

10. Bake for about 9 to 12 minutes until the calzones turn a light brown.

11. Use the pizza sauce when serving.

12. You will get 4 servings.

Nutritional Information (per serving)

- Calories- 264

- Fat- 8 g

- Saturated fat- 2 g

- Sodium- 590 mg

- Cholesterol- 8 mg

- Carbohydrate- 36 g

- Protein- 12 g

Vegetarian Tofu Chili

Number of Servings: 4

Ingredients

- Yellow onion- 1, chopped

- Olive oil- 1 tbsp

- Tomatoes- 2 cans of 14 ounces, no salt, diced

- Tofu- 12 ounces, firm, make pieces

- Black beans- 1 can of 14 ounces, no salt, rinse and drain

- Kidney beans- 1 can of 14 ounces, no salt, rinse and drain

- Oregano- 1 tbsp

- Chili powder- 3 tbsp

- Fresh cilantro- 1 tbsp, chopped

Steps to Cook

1. Use a large pot to heat some oil, keeping the heat medium.

2. Add the onions and cook to get a translucent texture in about 5 to 7 minutes.

3. Add the tomatoes, tofu, chili powder, beans and oregano. Boil, then simmer for about 35 to 40 minutes.

4. Remove from heat, and mix in the cilantro.

5. Serves 4 people.

Nutritional Information (per serving)

- Calories- 314

- Fat- 7 g

- Saturated fat- 0.9 g

- Sodium- 364 mg

- Cholesterol- 0 mg

- Carbohydrate- 46 g

- Protein- 19 g

Snacks and Beverages for a DASH Diet

Cinnamon Fruit Brie Packets

Number of Servings: 12

Ingredients

- Orange- 1/2, quartered

- Frozen cranberries- ½ cup, no salt

- Cinnamon- 1 stick

- Sugar- 2 tbsp

- Brie cheese- 6 ounces, cubed

- Pastry dough- 1 sheet, square cut pieces

- Egg white- 1

- Water- 2 tbsp

Steps to Cook

1. Preheat your oven to 425 degrees F.

2. During this time, heat a greased sauté pan, keeping the heat medium-high, and then reduce the heat, and put the orange, cranberries, cinnamon and sugar in to cook for about 8 to 9 minutes. Keep stirring the mixture

to make a consistent and thick sauce. Set aside to cool down, and then get rid of the orange quarters and the cinnamon stick.

3. In each puff pastry square, put in a cheese cube and the cranberry mixture.

4. Use a mixture of the water and egg white to seal the pastry squares in the shape of a diamond packet roll.

5. Coat the rolls with the rest of the egg white mixture and move to your baking dish.

6. Bake about 11 to 14 minutes to get the golden texture of the packets.

7. You will get 12 servings.

Nutritional Information (per serving)

- Calories- 116

- Fat- 6 g

- Saturated fat- 3 g

- Sodium- 133 mg

- Cholesterol- 22 mg

- Carbohydrate- 9 g

- Protein- 4 g

Parmesan and Basil Stuffed Mushrooms

Number of Servings: 5

Ingredients

- Crimini mushrooms- 20, wash and remove stems

- Melted butter- ¼ cup

- Breadcrumbs- 1 ½ cups, panko

- Parsley- 3 tbsp, freshly chopped

- Parmesan cheese- ¼ cup

- Basil leaves- 2 cups

- Olive oil- 1 tbsp

- Pumpkin seeds- 2 tbsp

- Lemon juice- 2 tsp

- Fresh garlic- 1 tbsp

- Kosher salt- ½ tsp

Steps to Cook

1. Preheat your oven to a temperature of 350 degrees F.

2. Take a baking dish and place mushrooms inside, keeping them upside down.

3. In a small-sized bowl, mix the butter, panko and parsley. Set aside.

4. Prepare the filling by combining the cheese, basil, pumpkin seeds, lemon juice, oil, salt and garlic. Blend this mixture in your food processor until it is the desired consistency.

5. Stuff the mushrooms with the prepared filling, and top with more panko.

6. Pat and bake for about 12 to 16 minutes.

7. You will get 20 golden brown stuffed mushrooms.

Nutritional Information (per serving)

- Calories- 59

- Fat- 2 g

- Saturated fat- 1.5 g

- Sodium- 80 mg

- Cholesterol- 7 mg

- Carbohydrate- 4 g

- Protein- 2 g

Cranberry Lemon Spritzer

Number of Servings: 4

Ingredients

- Lemon juice- ½ cup

- Cranberry juice- 1 quart, low-calorie

- Sugar- ¼ cup

- Carbonated water- 1 quart

- Lime wedges- 10

- Raspberry sherbet- 1 cup

Steps to Cook

1. Put the lemon juice and cranberry juice, as well as the carbonated water, in your refrigerator until cold.

2. In a large pitcher, mix all the juices along with the carbonated water, sherbet and sugar.

3. Pour into glasses and serve with lime wedges.

Nutritional Information (per serving)

- Calories- 60

- Fat- 0 g

- Saturated fat- 0 g

- Sodium- 20 mg

- Cholesterol- 0 mg

- Carbohydrate- 3 g

- Protein- 0.1 g

Mix Fruit Yogurt Kebabs

Number of Servings: 2

Ingredients
- Lime juice- 1 tsp, fresh

- Lemon yogurt- 6 ounces, sugar-free, low-fat

- Pineapple chunks- 4

- Lime zest- 1 tsp

- Kiwi- 1, peel and cut into quarters

- Strawberries- 4

- Red grapes- 4

- Banana- 1/2, into chunks

- Skewers- 4, wooden

Steps to Cook
1. In a small bowl, mix the lime juice and zest with yogurt. Cover the bowl to refrigerate.

2. Thread one piece of every fruit through the

wooden skewers.

3. Serve with the prepared yogurt and lemon dip.

   You will get 2 servings.

Nutritional Information (per serving)

- Calories- 190

- Fat- 2 g

- Saturated fat- 1 g

- Sodium- 53 mg

- Cholesterol- 5 mg

- Carbohydrate- 8 g

- Protein- 4 g

Ginger Blackberry Cold Tea

Number of Servings: 6

Ingredients

- Blackberry tea bags- 12, choose herbal ones

- Water- 6 cups

- Fresh ginger- 1 tbsp, minced

- Cinnamon- 8 sticks, 3 inch for each

- Sugar substitute- a little

- Cranberry juice- 1 cup, no sugar

- Ice cubes- enough for the tea, crushed

Steps to Cook

1. In a large saucepan, warm the water. Heat properly, but don't let it boil. Include the tea bags along with 2 sticks of cinnamon. Also, include the ginger and heat thoroughly.

2. Remove the pan from heat and cover. Leave this for about 14 to 17 minutes.

3. Transfer the mixture through a sieve, ensuring that the liquid goes into a pitcher. Include the sweetener and juice.

4. Refrigerate until cold and serve in 6 glasses with crushed ice. Garnish with the rest of the cinnamon sticks.

Nutritional Information (per serving)

- Calories- 30

- Fat- 0 g

- Saturated fat- 0 g

- Sodium- 3 mg

- Cholesterol- 0 mg

- Carbohydrate- 7 g

- Protein- 0 g

Tangy Melon, Pineapple and Strawberry Smoothie

Number of Servings: 2

Ingredients

- Cantaloupe melon- ½ cup
- Pineapple- 1 cup
- Oranges- 2, juiced
- Strawberries- 1 cup
- Honey- 1 tbsp
- Water- 1 cup

Steps to Cook

1. Cut the melon and pineapple into chunks.
2. Cut the strawberries into pieces after removing the stems.
3. Refrigerate all these ingredients until cold.
4. Blend all the ingredients together to make a puree in your food processor or blender.
5. Serve.

Nutritional Information (per serving)

- Calories- 72
- Fat- 0 g

- Saturated fat- 0 g

- Sodium- 8 mg

- Cholesterol- 0 mg

- Carbohydrate- 17 g

- Protein- 1 g

Conclusion

An optimal healthy life requires continuous management of what you eat. The DASH diet controls your sugar and sodium content and provides proper nutrition for your body. As a result, you lose weight, and get control of any hypertension.

Even if you have managed your weight and controlled hypertension, the DASH diet will allow you to stay that way your whole life.

However, it all comes down to how determined and consistent you are with the DASH diet, so keep following the knowledge and recipes in this book to stay healthy and manage your body weight.

Eat healthy, live healthy!

Sign-up to Get Our Next Book

for Free!

https://lizard-publishing.weebly.com

One Last Thing... Did You Enjoy the Book?

If so, then let me know by leaving a review on Amazon!
Reviews are the lifeblood of independent authors. I would appreciate even a few words from you!

If you did not like the book, then please tell me! Email me at lizard.publishing@gmail.com and let me know what you didn't like. Perhaps I can change it. In today's world, a book doesn't have to be stagnant. It should be improved with time and feedback from readers like you. You can impact this book, and I welcome your feedback. Help me make this book better for everyone!

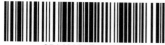

Made in the USA
Middletown, DE
24 October 2018